Clinical Bacteriology

CHURCHILL LIVINGSTONE MEDICAL TEXTS

Epidemiology in Medical Practice
Second Edition
D. J. P. Barker and G. Rose

Pain: Its Nature, Analysis and Treatment
Michael R. Bond

Elements of Medical Genetics
Fifth Edition
Alan E. H. Emery

Tumours: Basic Principles and Clinical Aspects
Christopher Louis

The Essentials of Neuroanatomy
Third Edition
G. A. G. Mitchell and D. Mayor

Sexually Transmitted Diseases
Third Edition
C. B. S. Schofield

Child Psychiatry for Students
Second Edition
Frederick H. Stone and Cyrille Koupernik

Notes on Medical Virology
Sixth Edition
Morag C. Timbury

Clinical Pharmacology
Third Edition
P. Turner and A. Richens

Immunology: An Outline for Students of Medicine and Biology
Fourth Edition
D. M. Weir

Clinical Thinking and Practice: Diagnosis and Decision in Patient Care
H. J. Wright and D. B. MacAdam

LIVINGSTONE MEDICAL TEXTS

Geriatric Medicine for Students
J. C. Brocklehurst and T. Hanley

An Introduction to Clinical Rheumatology
William Carson Dick

Physiology: A Clinical Approach
Second Edition
G. R. Kelman

A Concise Textbook of Gastroenterology
M. J. S. Langman

Introduction to Clinical Examination
Second Edition
Edited by John Macleod

Nutrition and its Disorders
Second Edition
Donald S. McLaren

An Introduction to Primary Medical Care
David Morrell

Urology and Renal Medicine
Second Edition
J. B. Newsam and J. J. B. Petrie

Psychological Medicine for Students
John Pollitt

Respiratory Medicine
Malcolm Schonell

An Introduction to General Pathology
W. G. Spector

Introduction to Clinical Endocrinology
John A. Thomson

Cardiology for Students
Max Zoob

Clinical Bacteriology

P. W. Ross

TD MD(Aberd)

Senior Lecturer, Department of Bacteriology,
University of Edinburgh Medical School, and
Honorary Consultant Bacteriologist,
Royal Infirmary, Edinburgh

Foreword by

B. P. Marmion

DSc MD FRCPath

Clinical Professor (Virology),
University of Adelaide
Director, Division of Virology,
Institute of Medical and Veterinary Science,
Adelaide, Australia
Formerly Professor of Bacteriology,
University of Edinburgh Medical School

CHURCHILL LIVINGSTONE
EDINBURGH LONDON AND NEW YORK 1979

CHURCHILL LIVINGSTONE
Medical Division of Longman Group Limited

Distributed in the United States of America by Churchill Livingstone Inc., 19 West 44th Street, New York, N.Y. 10036, and by associated companies, branches and representatives throughout the world.

ISBN 0 443 01811 1

British Library Cataloguing in Publication Data
Ross, P W
Clinical bacteriology.
1. Bacteriology, Medical
I. Title
616.01'4 QR46 79-40122

Printed in Singapore by Singapore Offset Printing Pte Ltd

Foreword

There are, broadly speaking, two ways of teaching about diseases produced by bacteria, viruses or other infective agents. One can start from the microorganism as such and proceed to the range of infections it produces. These may include different diseases in different body systems, or even some in different hosts: the organism represents the unity, the disease the diversity.

Alternatively, one can take a clinical condition at a single site (e.g., a sore throat), or in a single body system, and consider the diversity of infective agents that may produce closely similar clinical and pathological effects.

The latter 'syndrome' approach is probably more difficult for the student. It is, however, more closely related to the actual clinical situation in which the doctor has to review the possible causes of a suspected infection at a particular anatomical site in order to decide on confirmatory laboratory investigations, and initial chemotherapy.

The two approaches are not, of course, mutually exclusive. During the last ten years in Edinburgh we have placed more emphasis on the second, 'systems'-based approach, partly because of its greater clinical relevance and partly in an attempt to align our teaching with that of our colleagues in the clinical and pathological fields. Our students, however, have repeatedly pointed out the difficulty that most textbooks of microbiology are written in terms of organisms, rather than diseases.

In writing *Clinical Bacteriology* Dr Philip Ross has produced a text orientated to systems-based teaching that should fill a gap in the range of existing books and be of much value to medical and dental students.

Apart from refining and greatly extending departmental material used in the systems-based teaching and in the guide to the use of bacteriological and virological laboratories in the Royal Infirmary, Edinburgh, Dr Ross has added valuable sections on epidemiology and chemotherapy. The book should provide the clinician with a useful, quick guide to the range of potential pathogens to be expected at various anatomical sites and to the choice and methods of collection of specimens, in addition to chemotherapeutic possibilities.

B. P. M.

Preface

This book aims to provide the essentials of clinical bacteriology for those involved in the diagnosis and management of the infected patient, including medical and dental students, hospital medical staff and general practitioners. To help clarify the approach to problems of infection the different systems of the body have been dealt with in separate chapters; the clinical illness or lesion is the centre of focus rather than the organisms that cause it. Scientific details have been kept to a minimum as there are many excellent books available that can provide such information.

The text deals almost exclusively with bacterial infections, but as the diagnosis of infections must encompass a global microbiological approach, a list of the potential pathogens of each system is given in the figures at the beginning of the systems' chapters. Viruses, rickettsiae, chlamydiae, mycoplasmas, fungi and protozoa are included in these.

I have refrained from appending a list of antibiotics that may be used in the treatment of the various infections, except for a few instances where there are certain incontrovertible choices, or where it is likely that 'blind' therapy may have to begin without delay because of the seriousness of the infection. There is no place for guesswork in antimicrobial chemotherapy; bacteriological diagnosis with subsequent sensitivity testing must be performed.

In compiling this book I have consulted some of the material prepared and used in the medical and dental teaching of the Department of Bacteriology, University of Edinburgh, largely produced under the former headship of Professor B. P. Marmion and the current headship of Professor J. G. Collee, and I am grateful to them for permission to make use of it.

Several colleagues have been of great assistance to me in providing critical comments on the text and in checking the material. They are Dr Rex S. Miles, Dr John F. Peutherer, Dr W. A. Telfer Brunton and Mr Chris G. Cumming, Department of Bacteriology, University of Edinburgh; Dr Brian Watt and Dr W. Peter Holbrook, Central

Microbiological Laboratories, Western General Hospital, Edinburgh; Dr Ross St C. Barnetson, Department of Dermatology, University of Edinburgh; Mr Michael F. Smith, Royal Infirmary, Edinburgh; and Dr John G. Donald, Royal Infirmary, Perth. I am particularly indebted to Dr Miles for additions to the text.

My thanks are also due to Mr Ian Lennox and Miss Grace Foster, University of Edinburgh, for providing the illustrations, to Mrs Vivien McGrath for typing the script, to Dr Valerie Inglis for compiling the index, to Mrs Stella Ross for providing secretarial assistance and for checking the text and to Mr George W. Ross and Mrs Sylvia Ross for reading the proofs.

Finally, I wish to accord my appreciation to the staff of Churchill Livingstone for continued support during the compilation of this book.

Edinburgh, 1979 P. W. R.

Contents

1

Sources and spread of infections

Definitions

The terms *source*, *reservoir* and *vehicle* of infections are frequently confused and misused. *Source* refers to the *habitat* or growth area in the human or animal. *Reservoir* and *vehicle* refer to objects that are contaminated or colonised by microorganisms. For example, fingers may be the vehicle or reservoir for staphylococci derived from the anterior nares; milk may be the reservoir of *Brucella* organisms the source of which can be an infected cow and water may act as a reservoir for cholera vibrios whose source is the human intestine.

Infections may be *endogenous* (autogenous) or *exogenous*. *Endogenous infections* are contracted from the host himself. Many areas of the body have a normal, commensal flora characteristic of the particular area. A most important entity, this flora has many functions including the provision of a barrier to infection in the individual. Normally the organisms that comprise the commensal flora do not cause infection in the host but there are exceptions to the rule.

For example, two species of the viridans streptococci, *Streptococcus sanguis* and *mitis*, may produce infection in previously damaged heart valves when they enter the bloodstream from the mouth following dental extraction. *Streptococcus faecalis* can cause *infective endocarditis* and the source of these organisms is usually the urinary tract and intestine of the host. Their presence in the blood and consequently the heart valves may be the result of diagnostic surgical procedures such as cystoscopy. Other examples of endogenous infection include osteomyelitis in which *Staphylococcus aureus* may have been derived from a septic lesion in the skin; infection of burns by beta-haemolytic streptococci from the patient's own upper respiratory tract and urinary tract infection by *Escherichia coli* derived from the intestine. There are three common features in endogenous infections. Firstly, the infections are produced some distance away from the normal habitat of the organisms; secondly, such infections are frequently a manifestation of lowered tissue resistance or tissue damage; and finally, problems of endogenous infections are generally confined to the patient, in that they do not generally constitute high cross-infection risks.

Exogenous infections represent the greater proportion of infections and are derived from *Man*, *Animals* or the *Soil*. *Man* is the most common source of exogenous infection, either when the patient is suffering from *clinical infection* or when the person is a *carrier* of infection. In whooping cough, smallpox and influenza where the carrier state is thought not to exist, or at least to be of minimal importance in the transmission of infection, the clinical case is the source and such patients represent a major danger in the spread of these infections. The *incubation period* of an infection, weeks, days or hours before the clinical signs appear, is a dangerous period because the organisms are then actively multiplying in the organs and tissues.

Infections are commonly contracted from *carriers* and various types of these are described, such as *healthy*, *convalescent* and *chronic*. *Healthy carriers* harbour organisms in their tissues without showing any signs of clinical infection and because of this they constitute a particularly dangerous form of carrier. Streptococcal sore throat, various types of pneumonia and meningococcal meningitis can be contracted thus, as can intestinal infections such as bacillary dysentery and the enteric fevers. *Contact carriers* are those who acquire the infecting organisms from a patient but who do not become clinically ill. They may well have latent or subclinical infection and this can be identified by raised antibody titres in the serum; in outbreaks of poliomyelitis they may greatly outnumber the overt clinical cases in a community. *Paradoxical carriers* are those who acquire organisms from a carrier. *Convalescent carriers* are those who

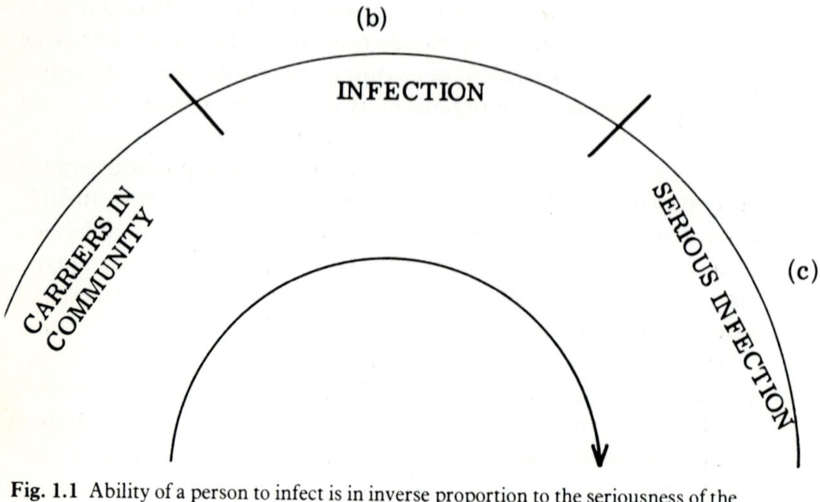

Fig. 1.1 Ability of a person to infect is in inverse proportion to the seriousness of the infection

shed organisms for variable periods after clinical infection. There is no defined period for convalescent carriage. Studies have shown that after an attack of diphtheria organisms persist in the throat of the patient for a period of several weeks, whereas after an attack of bacillary dysentery the carrier state can remain for several months. Administration of antimicrobial agents has frequently little or no effect in shortening the duration of carriage and in the case of intestinal infection may actually increase the duration. There is no clear-cut line of demarcation between the end of convalescent and the beginning of *chronic carriage*. In the case of typhoid fever, however, it is customary to describe carriage as chronic when more than one year has elapsed since the onset of the acute infection. In general terms much has still to be learned about the dynamics of the carrier state.

The ability of an individual to spread infection in a community is frequently in inverse proportion to the seriousness of the infection (Fig. 1.1).

Figure 1.1 (a) *Carriers in the community* are usually healthy, undetected and free to disseminate their organisms; (b) an infected, ill patient will contact his doctor who will either treat him at home or send him to hospital; he is *identified* as a case of infection. Alternatively, he may not seek medical help but he may at least stay off work or school; (c) in the case of *serious infection* the patient will be *isolated* in hospital, and will have special nursing and other procedures; the risks of spread of infection are then minimal.

Animals are also sources of infection that may be transmitted to man; such infections are known as *Zoonoses*. Spread of these is usually from animal to animal with the occurrence of an occasional human infection. In these cases the human is generally an *end-host* and does not further spread the infection except in rare instances such as pneumonic plague.

Examples of some diseases that can be acquired from animals can be seen in Table 1.1.

Soil has also a role in the production of infections. This is particularly so in infections with *Clostridium tetani* and *Clostridium welchii* in which soil is the reservoir rather than the source of infection; the source is generally the intestine of animals and the organisms gain access to the soil from animal faeces. Various fungal groups such as *Histoplasma* and *Microsporum* are also present in soil.

OUTBREAKS OF INFECTIONS

Infections in humans may be *endemic*, *epidemic* or *pandemic*.

Endemic infections are those normally present in a small proportion of the community and in the United Kingdom bacillary dysentery is a

Table 1.1 Infections that may be acquired from animals, birds and fish

Human disease	Organism	Principal sources
Anthrax	*Bacillus anthracis*	Cattle, goats, sheep
Brucellosis	*Brucella abortus, suis, melitensis*	Cattle, goats, pigs, sheep
Bacterial food infections and intoxications	Certain clostridia, salmonellae, *Staphylococcus aureus*	Cattle, pigs, poultry
Cryptococcosis	*Cryptococcus neoformans*	Cattle
Erysipeloid	*Erysipelothrix rhusiopathiae*	Fish, poultry, rodents
Lassa fever	Arenavirus	Mammals
Leptospirosis	*Leptospira canicola* and *icterohaemorrhagiae*	Dogs, pigs, rodents
Listeriosis	*Listeria monocytogenes*	Birds, mammals
Lymphocyticchoriomeningitis	Arenavirus	Mice and hamsters
Marburg disease	Marburg virus	African green monkeys
Plague	*Yersinia pestis*	Rats
Psittacosis	Chlamydia	Birds (parrots and pigeons)
Q fever	*Coxiella burneti*	Cattle, goats, sheep
Rabies	Rhabdovirus	Bats, dogs and carnivores (foxes)
Ratbite fever	*Spirillum minus, Streptobacillus moniliformis*	Rats
Ringworm	*Microsporum canis,*	Cats, dogs
	Trichophyton verrucosum	Cattle
Schistosomiasis	*Schistosoma japonicum*	Cattle, dogs, rodents
Tapeworm infection	*Taenia* spp	Cattle, pigs
Toxocariasis	*Toxocara canis*	Dogs
Toxoplasmosis	*Toxoplasma gondii*	Birds, mammals
Trypanosomiasis	*Trypanosoma* spp	Wild mammals
Tuberculosis	*Mycobacterium bovis*	Cattle
Yellow fever	Togavirus	Monkeys

good example of this. The endemic nature of infectious diseases depends on general factors such as social and economic conditions, on environmental factors such as population density and movement, standards of hygiene and sanitation and on general herd immunity. Generally herd immunity can be kept at a satisfactory level by immunisation procedures, as for example with measles, but clinical and subclinical infections are also important factors. *Exotic* infections are those that occur in endemic fashion and can be attributed to introduction of the disease from other countries. Cholera in the United Kingdom is such an example.

Epidemic infections result from any significant increase in the usually low incidence of endemic infections in a community. Many present-day epidemics particularly of virus infections such as influenza, measles and poliomyelitis are periodic. This periodicity is partly accounted for by an increase in the number of susceptible persons in the community, as may occur when vaccination rates fall. Epidemics may also be caused by a breakdown in hygiene, a change in the virulence of existing organisms, or the introduction to the community of a new organism as in Fiji in 1875 when the island's first epidemic of measles caused 20 000 deaths.

An epidemic that has reached massive proportions is described as a *pandemic*, for example the Asian influenza pandemic of 1957, and becomes a national or international rather than a community problem. Such outbreaks spread quickly from country to country.

When reference is made to infections in animal populations the terms *enzootic* rather than endemic, and *epizootic* rather than epidemic are used.

THE SPREAD OF INFECTIONS

There are four main routes by which a host may become infected: the respiratory tract; the alimentary tract; the skin and mucosae; and the placenta.

Spread of infections by the respiratory tract

Organisms that produce specific respiratory tract infections such as pneumonia enter the body by this route, as well as organisms that cause generalised systemic infections such as chickenpox and measles. Three main methods are recognised in the spread of respiratory tract infections: *contact*; *direct airborne*; and *indirect airborne*.

Contact

This can be direct or indirect. In *direct* contact such as kissing, infected droplets are passed from person to person; this is an important means of spread of respiratory pathogens that are poorly viable outside the body. For example, in whooping cough the secondary attack rate in families where contact is intimate may be as high as 90 per cent, whereas in less intimate situations such as in hospital wards the secondary attack is much lower. In *indirect* contact, organisms are transferred from inanimate reservoirs of infection (fomites) such as cups and eating utensils. Although the division is made into direct and indirect contact to distinguish between direct droplet spread from an infected person and the spread from an inanimate reservoir of infection, it is frequently impossible to tell which has been the means of transfer of organisms to the susceptible host.

Direct airborne spread

Droplets are expelled from the mouth in talking and coughing and to a much greater extent in sneezing, and are conveniently classified as *large* and *small droplets*. They are derived mostly from the saliva and only a proportion will be infected. *Large droplets* have a diameter of over 100 μm and having been expelled from the mouth fall quickly to the ground and on to surfaces and clothing. Most fall within six feet of the person. *Small droplets*, less than 100 μm in diameter, constitute the main part of the droplet mass. They evaporate rapidly and become minute solid secretions with a diameter of 5–10 μm, called *droplet nuclei*, that may or may not contain organisms. These particles being light can remain suspended in air currents for many hours and are probably the means of spread of many virus infections (Fig. 1.2).

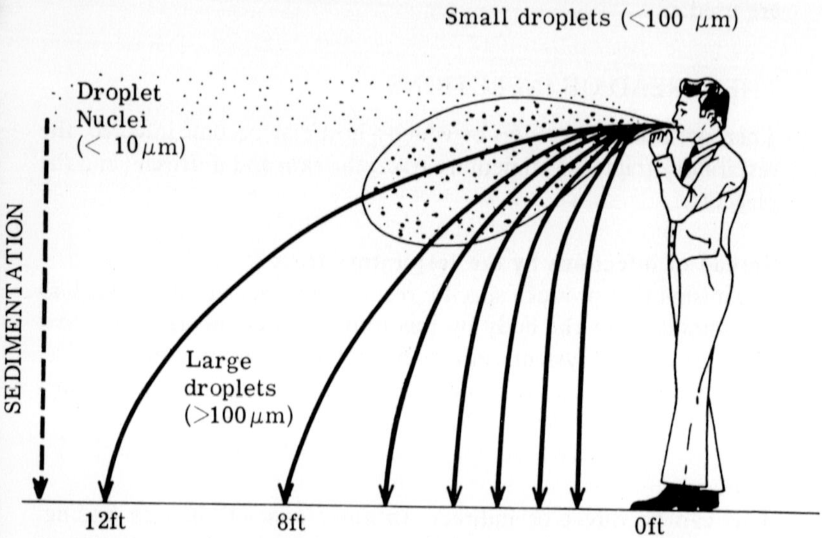

Fig. 1.2 Spread of droplets and droplet nuclei from the respiratory tract

Although droplet nuclei are considered important in the transmission of certain virus infections the role of the larger particles in producing direct airborne infection is less clear. Their importance may lie in their ability to contaminate the environment.

Indirect airborne spread

When large respiratory droplets fall from the air they land on exposed surfaces, clothing and floors and become dried particles of secretions in the dust. Some of these will be infectious secretions and if protected from sunlight organisms will remain viable for weeks or months. *Mycobacterium tuberculosis* and *Streptococcus pyogenes* are good examples of this and these organisms can be released into the air by activities such as sweeping, dusting and bedmaking. Also, when a handkerchief is shaken dried particles of potentially infectious secretions are released into the air.

Whereas there may be one main mode of spread for most infections other routes may be responsible from time to time. For example, transmission of beta-haemolytic streptococci that cause sore throat may be by direct contact, indirect contact from fingers or clothing, or by dust. Very occasionally respiratory infection, for example streptococcal sore throat, can be spread by consuming contaminated food and some cases of diphtheria have been attributed to drinking infected milk.

Spread of infections by the alimentary tract

The intestinal diseases, cholera, bacillary dysentery, the enteric fevers and bovine tuberculosis, are contracted when organisms are ingested, but the alimentary tract is also the route of entry of organisms such as enteroviruses, infectious hepatitis virus and *Brucella* spp whose effects are produced in other parts of the body.

Food contamination

Food may be contaminated at source or at any stage of its manufacture, preparation or storage. Contamination at source is exemplified by the infection of milk from a cow suffering from *Brucella* infection.

In the preparation of food, such as cream cakes, trifles and processed meat, organisms from many diverse sources can produce contamination. *Staphylococcus aureus* from the nose and skin of food handlers and *Salmonella* spp from hands, rodents and flies are but two examples. The symptomless carrier of salmonellae who is also a food handler is a dangerous source of infection. Milk is another potential danger particularly if it is not pasteurised. In the United Kingdom as much as 10–15 per cent is still unpasteurised in which case the individual runs the risk of infection by organisms such as *Brucella abortus*, *Streptococcus pyogenes*, salmonellae, staphylococci and *Coxiella burneti*.

Water contamination

Infections may result from drinking water contaminated by urine or faeces, water being the reservoir and not the source. In most areas of Europe piped-water supplies have largely abolished waterborne infections though there is a risk in areas not yet within reach of a public supply. Classical Asiatic cholera and typhoid fever are associated with transmission by water. The Aberdeen typhoid outbreak in 1964, although disseminated by contaminated canned corned beef, was really an example of a waterborne infection because water used in cooling the cans after their sterilisation was polluted with sewage and several cans were improperly sealed, resulting in the contamination of the meat.

Spread of infections by hands

This type of spread is the result of inadequate personal hygiene and the source is usually a carrier who contaminates his hands at defaecation; even a wad of several sheets of toilet paper may not be a barrier to organisms gaining access to the hands. These carriers contaminate toilet chains, wash basins, towels and door handles with their hands and infection is transmitted by another person putting his fingers to his mouth after handling contaminated articles. This is probably the means of spread of bacillary dysentery and poliomyelitis.

Spread of infections through the skin and mucosae

Simple contact

Some infections can be contracted through the skin and mucosae, for example the sexually transmitted diseases syphilis, gonorrhoea and lymphogranuloma venereum. The common wart, impetigo and ringworm can be similarly spread either by direct contact with the infected person or by contact with his clothing.

Contamination of wounds

A wound is taken as any breach of the surface of the skin and mucosae. Wounds resulting from trauma may be colonised by *Clostridium tetani*, particularly if contaminated by earth or dust. Abrasions and pricks by rose thorns can be similarly infected.

Sepsis of surgical wounds is one of the major infection problems of present-day hospitals and the causes of these are legion. A surgical wound is susceptible to infection from the moment of incision until it is completely healed and it is therefore exposed both in the operating theatre and in the ward. A vast literature has accumulated on wound sepsis in hospitals which highlights the roles of cases and carriers, operative and other surgical procedures, dressing techniques and environmental contamination in its production (Ch. 13).

Injection

Injection of organisms can result from *medical injections* and *animal* or *insect bites*.

Medical injection procedures, including blood transfusion, immunisation, prophylactic and therapeutic procedures, are seldom involved in the production of infection, although there is a well-known and very real risk of transmitting serum hepatitis by using needles contaminated with human blood. Outwith the medical field severe septicaemia can be caused in the drug addicts who make up their preparation for injection with unsterile water. A wide variety of organisms, including those of faecal origin, have been isolated from these.

Animal bites. Rabies and rat-bite fever are examples of infections introduced by animal bites, but many other organisms whose sources are animals can set up infection if the bite introduces them in sufficiently high numbers and if suitable conditions for multiplication are present.

Insect bites. Arthropods are important vectors of disease that in nature affect primarily animals and man only incidentally.

Table 1.2 indicates some vectors involved in the spread of disease to man.

Table 1.2 Vectors of disease

Fleas	:	bubonic plague
Lice	:	epidemic typhus; European relapsing fever; trench fever
Mites	:	rickettsial pox; scrub typhus
Mosquitoes	:	many infections including dengue, malaria and yellow fever
Ticks	:	African relapsing fever
Tsetse flies	:	trypanosomiasis

Spread of infections across the placenta

An uncommon route of spread, the only bacterial infection in which this has been clearly established is syphilis in which the infected mother transmits *Treponema pallidum*. Transplacental spread is more common in certain viral diseases, notably rubella and cytomegalovirus infection.

THE CONTROL OF SPREAD OF INFECTIONS

Although particular and specific measures can be applied to each infection, there are nevertheless general principles for the control and eradication of infections. These are:

Isolation or eradication of source

Isolation measures are useful in both humans and animals with clinical or suspected infections. Eradication of many bacterial infections is possible by the use of antimicrobial drugs. Removal of organisms by sterilisation procedures is routine in medical practice.

Blocking routes of spread

To control airborne infection is difficult although adequate ventilation of rooms and avoidance of overcrowding at times when respiratory diseases are prevalent may have some value. Formerly floors of hospitals and barracks were oiled to minimise infection from dust, but whether this was beneficial is open to doubt. Positive pressure ventilation in operating theatres, in isolation units and treatment rooms, has proved to be of value.

In the control of gastrointestinal diseases many measures can be taken, including maintaining purity of water supplies; ensuring pasteurisation of milk; maintaining scrupulous hygiene in the preparation and handling of food, together with bacteriological monitoring of food handlers and ensuring effective disposal of excreta.

Protection of susceptible individuals

Immunisation procedures have proved highly successful in the control of infections such as smallpox, poliomyelitis, diphtheria and tetanus. The administration of antimicrobial drugs may occasionally be useful in preventing certain infections in particularly susceptible individuals, for example the use of phenoxymethyl penicillin in the prevention of second attacks of rheumatic fever in children and adolescents. Great caution must be exercised however in administering antimicrobial drugs in the absence of firm bacteriological indications.

Finally, the resistance of patients to infection can be enhanced by general measures, for example the control of diabetes.

FURTHER READING

Burnet, F. M. (1962) *Natural History of Infectious Diseases*. Cambridge: Cambridge University Press.

Cruickshank, R., Duguid, J. P., Marmion, B. P. & Swain, R. H. A. (1973) *Medical Microbiology*. Edinburgh: Churchill Livingstone.

Dubos, R. J. & Hirsch, J. G. (1965) *Bacterial and Mycotic Infections of Man*. 4th edn. London: Pitman.

Passmore, R. & Robson, J. S. (1973) *A Companion to Medical Studies*. Vol. 2, revised reprint. Oxford: Blackwell Scientific Publications.

Wilson, G. S. & Miles, A. A. (1975) *Topley and Wilson's Principles of Bacteriology and Immunity*. 6th edn. London: Arnold.

2

Bacterial pathogenicity

PATHOGENS

Pathogens are microorganisms that can cause disease in man and animals. *True* pathogens are those which by virtue of their properties frequently produce infection when in the host, although this is not inevitable since the host may be immune to the infecting organism; there are many other factors involved in the host-pathogen relationship. *Opportunist* pathogens are those which do not cause infection in the normal course of events but which may infect the *compromised host* — the person who suffers from hormonal, metabolic or malignant disease and the patient who is receiving either cytotoxic drugs or steroid hormones. Those undergoing immunosuppressive therapy are also very susceptible to infection with a wide variety of organisms because of derangement of the normal defence mechanisms of the body.

Virulence

This is a measure of the pathogenicity of the organism. All pathogens are endowed with some degree of virulence which depends on many factors including *structural components*, such as capsules, and *diffusible products*. Successful attempts have been made to measure the virulence of organisms in animals and the minimum lethal dose (MLD) and median lethal dose (LD50) can be calculated. The MLD is ascertained by injecting serial dilutions of the organisms and finding the smallest dose required to kill the animal. As with humans however the resistance of animals can vary to a considerable extent and the LD50, or the dose required to kill approximately 50 per cent of the group of animals, may be a more useful measure of virulence. Death may not necessarily be the best criterion.

Infectivity

The *infectivity* of an organism is its pathogenic potential. This includes successful entry to the body, establishment in the tissues and exertion of its pathogenic effects through *invasiveness*, *toxigenicity* or a combination of both.

TRANSMISSIBILITY OF INFECTION

There are several factors involved in the transmission of infection from the original to the new host; for example, in the transmission of whooping cough close proximity to the original case is necessary. The *size of the infecting dose* is also important because successful transmission depends on having a sufficient number of organisms present to enter the body, overcome the host resistance and become established in the tissues. The dose of organisms required to initiate infection can be altered by certain factors such as the presence of foreign bodies in tissues and experiments have shown that the threshold number of organisms required to initiate a staphylococcal skin lesion can be reduced considerably from the several million required in normal circumstances if foreign bodies such as skin sutures are present.

Survival of organisms outside the body

This form of survival is important in the natural history of several infections. Spore-forming pathogens such as *Bacillus anthracis* and *Clostridium tetani* are notable for their survival outside the body, but more delicate organisms and strict parasites can survive for only limited periods under normal conditions.

Survival of organisms in immune individuals

This is an important factor particularly in infections such as typhoid in which the bacilli can localise in the biliary tract, and related to this is the situation where persons become carriers without ever having had the clinical illness.

Survival of organisms in vectors or intermediate hosts

Bubonic plague is spread by rat fleas and a critical factor in the chain of events leading to infection of new hosts is the ability of the plague bacilli to infect the fleas.

Events after the bacterial attack

Events depend largely upon the nature of the host-parasite association but the effects are essentially *localised* or *generalised*.

Localised infection

Many infections remain localised and only become generalised if the organism becomes more virulent, if the host resistance is decreased or if the bacteria gain access to another susceptible part of the body. The staphylococcal boil or furuncle typifies the localised infection, although many other bacteria can produce local lesions. Gonococci affect the urethra and conjunctiva and shigella organisms the intestinal mucosa.

Localised infection with diffusion of toxin

Diphtheria and streptococcal infections of the throat produce frank local infection with concomitant symptoms and signs as well as systemic involvement due to release of toxin. Other such infections include gas gangrene in which there may be only minimal local signs.

Generalised infection

Some organisms are highly invasive when they enter the body and produce a generalised infection. Some are classically acute as in the case of enteric fevers and others such as brucellosis may be subacute although acute episodes of the latter can occur. Spread can be direct, by the cerebrospinal fluid, by the blood or by lymphatics; certain organisms have a predilection for a particular organ or type of tissue, for example rabies virus and the central nervous system.

Direct spread

The outcome of this depends on the result of the host-parasite encounter. Organisms that spread in the skin and subcutaneous tissues are frequently those that produce factors that facilitate their spread, for example streptokinase in the case of streptococcal infections. The moisture on mucosal surfaces, such as in the intestine or urethra, is thought to play a part in spreading infection and establishing new foci in different areas.

Direct spread is not limited to skin and mucosal surfaces and there are many examples of direct spread within organs and tissues. In infection of the middle ear, for example, spread can occur to neighbouring structures such as the meninges and any focus of infection in the pelvis such as salpingitis can spread to involve the peritoneum. Similarly, pleurisy can result from an extension of lobar pneumonia.

Spread by the blood

This form of spread is an efficient means of disseminating organisms borne free in the plasma or within the white blood cells. Those carried free include staphylococci, streptococci and coliform organisms; such organisms are vulnerable to attack from the various defence mechanisms of the host. Bacteria carried by the white cells, particularly monocytes and lymphocytes, include *Brucella* spp and

Mycobacterium tuberculosis and these are largely protected from the host defence factors. *Bacteriaemia* is simply the presence of bacteria in the blood and is a common occurrence. It can be produced merely by brushing teeth, or chewing, or by diagnostic procedures such as sigmoidoscopy and urinary tract catheterisation. It is generally a transient phenomenon as the bacteria are not actively multiplying and are quickly removed by the action of the host defences. Conversely, when large numbers of bacteria enter the bloodstream and actively multiply a *septicaemia* is produced. This is quite different from a simple bacteriaemia because the patient is clinically ill, often with focal infection in some organ, and the infection will progress unless controlled by antimicrobial drugs, with or without surgical intervention.

Spread by lymphatics

Bacteria can invade the lymphatic system in almost any part of the body but in most cases the lymph glands draining the various areas filter off the organisms and prevent further spread centrally. Some particularly virulent bacteria may not be filtered off and killed by the lymph glands and may spread to other areas of the body; indeed, some organisms may multiply actively within the gland. Organisms that spread via the lymphatic system include *Mycobacterium tuberculosis*, *Yersinia pestis*, *Brucella* spp and *Salmonella typhi*.

Spread by the cerebrospinal fluid

Bacteria in the blood can enter the cerebrospinal fluid (CSF) through the choroid plexus of the ventricles. Once within the subarachnoid space organisms spread very quickly because the CSF is devoid of any effective antibacterial properties. *Neisseria meningitidis*, *Haemophilus influenzae*, pneumococci and *Mycobacterium tuberculosis* enter the CSF from the bloodstream although bacteria may also gain access directly, as in the case of trauma to the skull or congenital deformities of the spinal cord.

TOXIGENICITY

Bacterial toxins can be broadly divided into those secreted by bacteria during active growth, the *exotoxins*, and those associated with the structure of the organism such as the cell wall which are released after death of the cell, the *endotoxins*. Properties of toxins are shown in Table 2.1.

Table 2.1 represents the classical view of differentiation of the toxins but is not strictly accurate. For example, protein toxins of some

Table 2.1 A comparison of exotoxins and endotoxins

Exotoxins	Endotoxins
Produced by Gram-positive bacteria	Produced by Gram-negative bacteria
Protein	Lipopolysaccharide
Heat-labile	Heat-stable
Liberated from cytoplasm of multiplying bacteria	Liberated from cell wall of dead or disintegrating bacteria
Converted into toxoid by H.CHO	Cannot be toxoided
Highly specific for certain tissues	Non-specific
High potency	Low potency
Strongly antigenic	Poorly- or non-antigenic
Effectively neutralised by antitoxin	Not effectively neutralised by antitoxin

bacteria may be produced intracellularly as well as extracellularly during active growth and thus a new classification has been suggested, as shown in Table 2.2.

Table 2.2 Recent classification of bacterial toxins (Raynaud, M. & Alouf, J. E. (1970) *Microbial Toxins*, **1**, Ch. 3, p. 67)

Group 1:	Intracytoplasmic protein toxins of Gram-negative bacteria.
Group 2:	Endotoxins of cell walls of Gram-negative bacteria.
Group 3:	True protein exotoxins.
Group 4:	Protein toxins with both intracellular and extracellular location during logarithmic phase.

Exotoxins

These are produced by several groups of Gram-positive bacteria such as *Clostridium botulinum*, *Clostridium welchii* and *Clostridium tetani*, *Corynebacterium diphtheriae*, *Streptococcus pyogenes* and *Staphylococcus aureus* and Gram-negative bacteria such as *Shigella dysenteriae* and *Vibrio cholerae*. Many have affinities for particular tissues; for example, tetanus toxin affects the anterior columns of the spinal cord, diphtheria toxin the heart and peripheral nerve endings and staphylococcal toxin the vomiting centre in the central nervous system. Effects of toxins are *local* or *systemic*. Toxins acting locally include those produced by bacteria that gain access to the intestine by ingestion and exert their effect on small blood vessels and the intestinal mucosa, producing small ulcers as the result of toxic destruction of the epithelial cells. *Vibrio cholerae* releases a toxin that attaches to specific receptors on the epithelial cells, causing a rise in the level of cyclic adenosine monophosphate, thereby stimulating excessive secretion of water and electrolytes from the undamaged cells of the intestinal mucosa.

Exotoxins that exert their effects at a distance are produced by *Corynebacterium diphtheriae*, *Clostridium tetani* and *Streptococcus pyogenes*. There is some controversy as to whether the typical skin rash of scarlet fever is due to a primary effect of the erythrogenic toxins or whether it is a manifestation of a hypersensitivity reaction to the toxins.

Toxoid

This is toxin that has been treated with certain chemicals such as formalin resulting in a loss of toxicity without altering its antigenicity. A toxoid is a good antigen and produces antitoxic antibody in man.

Endotoxins

These are complex polysaccharide-protein-phospholipid molecules associated with the cell walls of Gram-negative bacteria including *Escherichia coli*, *Proteus* spp, salmonellae, shigellae and *Bacteroides* spp and they produce many toxic effects in the body, particularly in the vascular system, causing a drastic fall in blood pressure. They are also very powerful pyrogens.

Endotoxic shock

Shock is often associated with a Gram-negative septicaemia related to the release of endotoxin from the bacteria in the bloodstream. Whether Gram-negative or bacteriogenic shock is synonymous with endotoxic shock is doubtful as some patients suffer Gram-negative shock with no evidence of circulating endotoxin. In addition, a syndrome similar to endotoxic shock can be caused by organisms that do not possess endotoxin. There may be some overlap in the causes of bacteriogenic and endotoxic shock although separate mechanisms may operate for each; the results are clinically similar, and many clinicians use the term 'septic shock'.

Patients with bacteriogenic or endotoxic shock are frequently those who have undergone a diagnostic procedure such as instrumentation of the urinary tract or they may have an active infection in the form of urinary tract infection or cholecystitis. Non-septic patients such as those who have suffered burns or trauma may be similarly affected.

Endotoxins may be detected in the blood of patients after instrumentation of the urinary tract with no subsequent deleterious effects and clinical manifestations may therefore be dose-related; the dramatic effects on the vascular system may occur only after large amounts of endotoxin enter the bloodstream. In addition to the effects on the vascular system by way of peripheral vascular pooling, drastic fall in blood pressure, collapse and possible death, endotoxin can be a cause of intravascular thrombosis. The condition is known as *disseminated intravascular coagulation* and is the result of clumping of the red blood cells consequent to an increase in capillary permeability and loss of fluid from the vascular system, together with activation of the blood clotting mechanism.

INVASIVENESS

The capacity of bacteria to invade, become established and multiply in tissues is an important aspect of bacterial pathogenicity, and is typically associated with pneumococci, *Mycobacterium tuberculosis* and *Brucella* spp.

Other organisms such as *Neisseria gonorrhoeae* are not markedly invasive yet remain successful pathogens.

AGGRESSINS

Whether they produce infection by toxigenicity, invasiveness or a combination of both, bacteria possess structural components and other factors in the cytoplasm that contribute to the production of infection. These substances such as collagenases are not pathogenic in their own right but may nevertheless promote the pathogenicity of the organism. Factors that promote the initiation and spread of infection are often termed '*aggressins*', whether or not they themselves possess any toxic activity. Examples of aggressins are as follows:

Surface components

Prominent amongst these are bacterial *capsules*. Pneumococci possess polysaccharide capsules that help resist phagocytosis and the action of bactericidal substances in the body fluids; on the other hand, antibodies to these capsules assist phagocytosis and protect against infection. Other capsulate organisms are *Klebsiella pneumoniae* and *Haemophilus influenzae*.

Other surface components include the non-antigenic hyaluronic acid capsule of *Streptococcus pyogenes* but this is less effective in protection against phagocytosis than another surface component, the M-protein. Certain Gram-negative bacilli, particularly the enterobacteriaciae, form a layer of acidic polysaccharide outside their cell walls, which although not sufficiently substantial to be termed a capsule has nevertheless certain antiphagocytic properties.

Diffusible products

Many diffusible products in addition to the exotoxins can act as aggressins.

Hyaluronidase

Sometimes known as the *spreading factor* this is produced by *Staphylococcus aureus*, beta-haemolytic streptococci and *Clostridium welchii*. It acts by breaking down the intercellular hyaluronic acid that binds cells together, allows spread of bacteria through the tissues and is thought to be important in the initiation of infection. There are anomalies in that *Staphylococcus aureus* produces large amounts but invasiveness and spread are not the hallmarks of typical staphylococcal skin infection and in infection by *Clostridium welchii* antibodies to hyaluronidase neither prevent initiation of infection nor check its progress.

Coagulase

This substance is produced by *Staphylococcus aureus*. It is an enzyme that produces a fibrin envelope round the organisms conferring partial protection from phagocytosis. As yet no role has been found for coagulase in the production of infection and its usefulness may be more as a marker in the laboratory identification of pathogenic staphylococci.

Fibrinolysin

Some pathogenic staphylococci, groups A, C and G beta-haemolytic streptococci and *Bacteroides* spp produce this substance. A synonym for staphylococcal fibrinolysin is *staphylokinase* and for the streptococcal form *streptokinase*. The action of fibrinolysin may be to break down the protective fibrin barriers in areas of infected tissue and promote spread of the infection. Streptokinase is antigenic.

Collagenase

Several bacteria including *Bacteroides* and *Clostridium welchii* produce this substance. The latter possesses a powerful collagenase that has a destructive effect on various tissues including muscle but its role in pathogenicity is obscure; anticollagenase antibodies neither protect against nor limit the infection.

Neuraminidase

Produced by various bacteria this is a mucinase that catalyses the hydrolysis of mucoproteins at the cell surface and may render the cell more vulnerable to bacterial attack.

Lecithinase
An alpha-toxin is produced by *Clostridium welchii* which hydrolyses lecithin, with resulting lysis of erythrocytes and necrosis of cells.

Deoxyribonucleases (DNAses) (streptodornase)
These are important in groups A, C and G streptococci, and four distinct types, A–D, are found in *Streptococcus pyogenes*. Streptodornase and streptokinase can be used clinically to dissolve fibrinous exudates. Antibody response to DNAse B is common in patients with streptococcal infection.

Many bacteria produce a variety of substances that may or may not contribute to pathogenicity including amylases, esterases, lipases, mucinases and proteinases.

ADHERENCE

Bacterial adherence whether to smooth surfaces or to cells can be an important mechanism in the pathogenic process. Some viridans streptococci produce dextran and mutan from dietary carbohydrate and consequently can adhere to tooth surfaces; this adherence by acidogenic *Streptococcus mutans* may be the first step in the pathogenesis of dental caries. There are several examples of bacterial adherence to tissue cells and in these adherence would appear to be a prerequisite for colonisation which in turn may be a prerequisite for infection. Cholera vibrios adhere to intestinal cells, *Bordetella pertussis* to the ciliated epithelium of the upper resporatory tract and *Streptococcus pyogenes* to the pharyngeal mucosa. Lipoteichoic acid is of importance in binding certain bacteria to the membranes of epithelial cells.

FACTORS THAT PREDISPOSE TO INFECTION

Host factors

Age. Susceptibility to infection is greatest in the very young and the elderly and probably relates to the effectiveness of the inflammatory and immune responses.

Genetic factors are sometimes ill-defined, as in the susceptibility of certain races to tuberculosis and the occurrence of rheumatic fever in twins, but there is increasing belief that the immune response, which is under genetic control, is of importance. The *sex* of the host may be important; for example, the death rate from whooping cough in the first year of life is much higher in females, although exposure to the disease is equal with males. An explanation of sex differences may lie in hormonal influences.

Pre-existing disease. In burns, for example, one of the greatest threats to survival is overwhelming infection. Patients on steroids and immunosuppressive drugs and those with malignant disease are very susceptible to infection.

Environmental factors

Nutrition has for long been known to influence infections. In recent wars, for example, infections and other diseases were rife in prisoners who were deprived of proper nutrition. Little is known about why resistance should be lowered in malnutrition although protein deficiency is known to depress the cell-mediated immune response, producing for example a greater susceptibility to an infection such as tuberculosis. In addition, deficiencies of certain vitamins such as A and C have a deleterious effect on mucosal barriers.

Climate is important; for example, respiratory tract infections are more common in the winter months in the United Kingdom.

Animal contact. Veterinary surgeons run a high risk of brucellosis.

Local factors

Some areas of the body have very poor resistance to infection, for example the meninges, anterior chamber of the eye and joints. Other factors such as *surgical interference*, *poor blood supply* and the *presence of foreign bodies* all predispose to infection.

GENERAL HOST RESPONSES TO INFECTION

There are many local and general alterations in the host in response to infection other than phagocytosis and the immune response.

Fever

This is a regular feature of systemic infection and is thought to be the product of bacterial factors such as endotoxin, and host factors such as products of tissue injury. The pathogenesis of the mechanisms of production of fever is complex and may well be multifactorial.

Circulatory changes

Circulatory failure may be *central* or *peripheral*. Central or cardiac failure may occur as the result of damage to valves as in infective endocarditis or after damage to the mycocardium following diphtheria. Peripheral failure, or shock, characterised by events such as severe hypotension, hyperventilation, oliguria and tachycardia, can be caused by the septicaemic state and by endotoxins.

Haematological changes

Many systemic infections produce changes in the number and proportions of white cells. In pyogenic infections a polymorphonuclear leucocytosis occurs and in typhoid fever a leucopaenia.

Although many other changes are recognised, including muscle weakness, weight loss, electrolyte imbalance, increase in the basal metabolic rate and stimulation of the adrenal cortex, much has still to be learned about the basic physio-pathological changes that occur in the host as the result of infection.

Persistent infection

Some infections can persist for months or even years, as for example tuberculosis, in which bacteria can remain in lung or renal tissue or in a lymph gland, and typhoid fever in which the salmonellae persist in the gall-bladder. In certain instances organisms that persist can cause chronic disease and this is seen in tuberculosis and brucellosis.

FURTHER READING

Ajl, S. J., Ciegler, A., Kadis, S., Montie, T. C. & Weinbaum, G. (1970–1972) *Microbial Toxins*, (vols. I–V). London: Academic Press.

Cruickshank, R., Duguid, J. P., Marmion, B. P. & Swain, R. H. A. (1973) *Medical Microbiology*. Edinburgh: Churchill Livingstone.

Dubos, R. J. & Hirsch, J. G. (1965) *Bacterial and Mycotic Infections of Man*. London: Pitman.

Smith, H. & Pearce, J. H. (1972) *Microbial Pathogenicity in Man and Animals*. Cambridge: Cambridge University Press.

3

Prevention of infections

Various mechanisms protect the individual from infection. Some are non-specific like the mucus secretion of the ciliated epithelium of the upper respiratory tract, the high acidity of the gastric juice and the vagina, whereas others such as the formation of antibodies against pathogenic organisms are quite specific.

DEFENCES IN THE HOST

Innate immunity

The determinants of this are genetically controlled in that there may be a marked difference in the response of species and individuals to infecting organisms. Man is immune to many animal infections and *vice versa*. *Salmonella typhi* produces a serious infection in man and *Salmonella typhimurium* causes only a mild localising intestinal infection, whereas in mice the situation is reversed. Within species, Algerian sheep are resistant to anthrax whereas European sheep are highly susceptible, and similarly it is known that Indian and Pakistan immigrants to the United Kingdom are more susceptible to tuberculosis than Caucasians. Natural selection may play an important role in differences within species. Nutritional and hormonal factors as well as age may also have to be considered in the analysis of innate immunity.

Mechanical barriers

These will be mentioned only briefly here as they will be described in later chapters. Mechanical barriers to infection are essentially the intact skin and mucous membranes, the skin providing the more effective protection because of its outer horny layer. Joint synovia and muscle fascia also have a protective function.

Bacteriocidal secretions

Sebum, sweat, mucus, saliva, tears, gastric and intestinal juices act by washing bacteria off the various body surfaces. This effect can be supplemented by other defence mechanisms, for example the action of the cilia in the upper respiratory tract. Other bacteriocidal substances including various acids and bacteriocines, play a useful defensive role. The components of the *normal flora* of the various anatomical sites are largely responsible for preventing the establishment of new and possibly pathogenic organisms. The mechanisms involve antibacterial substances such as lactic acid produced by the lactobacilli in the vagina, hydrogen peroxide by the viridans streptococci in the mouth and propionic acid by the propionibacteria on the skin. The normal flora plays a key role in defence against infection and when this is suppressed by the administration of broad-spectrum antibiotics pathogenic bacteria can then invade the denuded areas much more easily. *Lysozyme*, present in most tissue fluids except urine, cerebrospinal fluid and sweat, has a mucolytic effect on the cell walls of many Gram-positive bacteria; glycopeptides are split off with subsequent lysis of the bacteria.

PHAGOCYTOSIS AND THE INFLAMMATORY RESPONSE

When bacteria successfully penetrate the body's non-specific barriers to infection and gain access to the tissues changes known as the *inflammatory response* occur. *Phagocytosis* is central to this. Phagocytes are white blood cells specialised to ingest and digest organisms. There are two types — (1) the neutrophil polymorphonuclear leucocytes (polymorphs) of the blood, the *microphages*, and (2) the large mononuclear phagocytic cells, the *macrophages*; these can either be freely circulating in the blood or fixed in the cells of the reticulo-endothelial system, the liver sinuses (Kuppfer cells), bone marrow, lymph glands and spleen. Macrophages in the blood are called *monocytes*, those in the connective tissues *histiocytes* and those in the lymph glands *reticulum cells*. In addition to dealing with bacteria phagocytes have also a role in removing other foreign material from the bloodstream.

When bacteria invade the body leucocytes leave the bloodstream and move towards the invaders. This is known as *chemotaxis* and operates as the result of production of chemical mediators at the site of infection. The leucocytes have then to bind to the bacteria, probably by electrostatic forces, before the organisms can be ingested and digested. Ingestion by the polymorphs occurs by an invagination of the cell membrane around the organisms and the organisms are enclosed in a vacuole formed by the cell membrane. After ingestion granules contained in the cytoplasm of the polymorphs, *lysozomes*, fuse with the vacuole containing the organisms and disappear. This disappearance is due to the discharge of their contents into the phagocytic vacuole and is triggered off by fusion of the membrane of the lysozome with that of the vacuole. The bacteriocidal substances liberated by the lysozome are lactic acid, lysozyme, phagocytin, phosphatases and ribonuclease. Most phagocytosed bacteria are digested within two hours, but *Mycobacterium tuberculosis* may survive for much longer periods and *Listeria monocytogenes* and *Brucella abortus* can survive and multiply within macrophages. Survival of certain species within phagocytes may be facilitated by their secretion of substances that are deleterious or lethal to the cells.

Bacteria that successfully avoid or survive phagocytosis are confronted by a further line of defences, the *immune system* of the body. When the bacteria are confronted by the cells of the immune system a specific immune response occurs. This response is in two forms, *humoral immunity* and *cell-mediated immunity*, which often develop in parallel and are dependent on lymphoid cells.

THE IMMUNE RESPONSE

The immune response or *humoral antibody* response, whether to natural infection or to immunisation procedures, has several well-defined features. After exposure to the antigen there is a *latent period* before antibody, mainly IgM, is detected in the blood; this period is around 10–14 days, during which time protein synthesis and cellular multiplication take place in the lymphoid tissues. When antibody is detected in the blood this is known as the *primary immune response* (Fig. 3.1). This response is characteristically *transient*, antibodies do not reach a high level and soon disappear. If however a second dose of antigen is given, a very marked rise in the level of antibody, mainly IgG, occurs, this time in only a few days. This is the *secondary response* (Fig. 3.2) and the level of antibody persists for considerably longer periods before falling off. If a further booster is given the antibody level rises sharply and persists for even longer periods. *Immunological memory* remains for years after initial contact of the antigen with the antibody-forming cells, and further contact at a much later date can result in continued production of high levels of antibody. Antibody is produced by *B lymphocytes*, derived from the liver in the foetus and from the bone marrow in the adult and differentiated into *plasma cells*.

Humoral immunity

This type of immunity is related to the presence in the bloodstream of *antibodies* or *immunoglobulins* which combine specifically with the

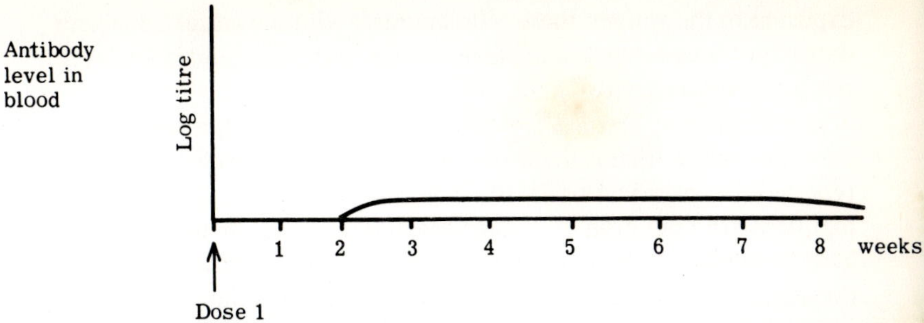

Fig. 3.1 Primary response

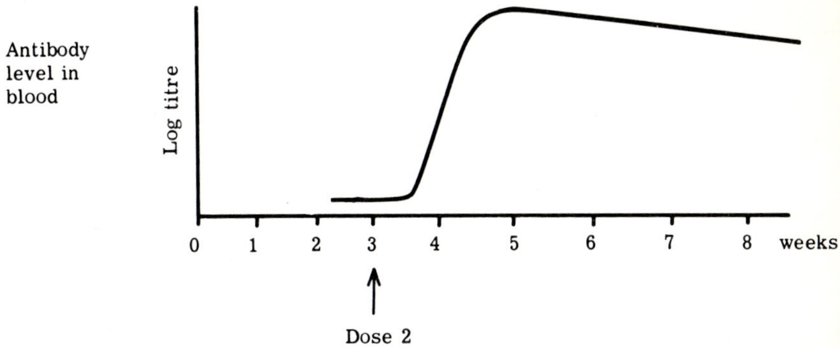

Fig. 3.2 Secondary response

antigen. Antibodies formed against an antigen include the three main immunoglobulin classes, *IgG*, *IgA* and *IgM*.

Antibodies have several antimicrobial actions: (1) they combine with bacterial surfaces and prevent attachment to susceptible mucosal surfaces; (2) they activate the complement system and promote phagocytosis of the antigen-antibody complex; and (3) they neutralise the effect of bacterial toxins.

Secretory immunoglobulins

IgA antibody is present in blood but is also present in a modified form in secretions in the respiratory and alimentary tracts. At these important routes of entry it may prevent infection. It is an important advantage of live vaccines that they can produce this form of protection.

Cell-mediated immunity (CMI)

T-lymphocytes (thymus-derived) generate CMI responses and are present both in the blood and lymphoid tissues. Having had previous exposure to the antigen these cells can react with the antigen at a later date to produce detrimental effects such as graft rejection and delayed tissue hypersensitivity.

In infections by *Mycobacterium tuberculosis* and *Brucella* spp there is reason to believe that cellular immunity of a delayed hypersensitivity type is the primary basis of acquired immunity. This can be highlighted in children with agammaglobulinaemia or hypogammaglobulinaemia. Although they may be resistant to infections with these intracellular bacteria, their resistance to infections with other organisms is considerably reduced. CMI is detectable in several infections by skin testing.

Acquired immunity

Active	Natural Artificial
Passive	Natural Artificial

Active natural immunity

This results either from a clinical or subclinical infection and is directed towards the organism that causes the infection. Some infections such as whooping cough and diphtheria produce long-lasting immunity, whereas in others such as gonorrhoea the period of immunity may be quite brief. It is worth noting that an attack of tetanus does not produce any immunity and an individual who has suffered the disease must be actively immunised to prevent future attacks.

Active artificial immunity

This results from immunisation procedures. It can be produced by injection of living attenuated organisms as in BCG vaccination against tuberculosis, by injection of killed organisms as in protection against whooping cough and the enteric fevers, and by administration of toxoid as used for the prophylaxis of tetanus and diphtheria.

Passive natural immunity.

This is produced in the foetus by transplacental IgG antibodies from the mother and means that the baby will have some form of minimal protection to certain infections for the first two or three months of life. Antibodies of the IgA class are also acquired in the first few weeks from the mother's milk.

Passive artificial immunity
Administration of immune serum which may be either human or prepared in another species such as the horse, and pooled human immunoglobulin, confer this form of transient immunity. There are dangers in giving heterologous antiserum because of the possibility of severe hypersensitivity reactions. Human immunoglobulin does not produce such effects and is safe to use, but nevertheless active immunisation is always preferable to passive because of its prolonged protection and comparative safety.

IMMUNISATION

The following are indications for immunisation:

1. Protection of members of a community in infancy or early life against potentially serious diseases that can occur in the community.
2. Protection of travellers going to countries where there are infections not prevalent in their own country.
3. Protection of nations or communities in the face of a possible epidemic.
4. Protection of groups at special risk, such as hospital personnel, the old and infirm, and those with debilitating diseases.

Vaccines

There are three forms of antigen used in immunisation procedures: (1) *Attenuated living*; (2) *Killed*, by chemicals such as formalin or alcohol; and (3) *Toxoids*, toxins that have been made non-toxic either by the action of heat or the addition of formalin.

Immunisation schedules (Table 3.1)

Vaccination against smallpox is no longer recommended as a routine procedure in the United Kingdom because of the almost complete eradication of smallpox throughout the world. It is vital however that hospital personnel and public health workers should be fully protected against the disease.

Complications of immunisation procedures

Smallpox
Local sepsis at the site of the vaccination and also more severe side effects such as eczema vaccinatum, post-vaccinial encephalitis and generalised vaccinia are possible.

Typhoid/paratyphoid
Fever, rigors and headache are common complications.

Table 3.1 Schedule of vaccination and immunisation procedures — 1972 — extracted with minor amendments from Memo. of Standing Medical Advisory Committee (HMSO, July, 1972)

Age	Vaccine	Interval	Notes
During the first year of life	Diph/Tet/Pert and oral polio vaccine. (First dose)		The earliest age at which the first dose should be given is 3 months, but a better general immunological response can be expected if the first dose is delayed to 6 months
	Diph/Tet/Pert and oral polio vaccine. (Second dose)	Preferably after an interval of 6 to 8 weeks.	
	Diph/Tet/Pert and oral polio vaccine. (Third dose)	Preferably after an interval of 4 to 6 months.	
During the second year of life	Measles vaccine	After an interval of not less than 3 weeks.	Although measles vaccination can be given in the second year of life, delay until the age of three years or more will reduce the risk of occasional severe reactions to the vaccine.
At 5 years of age or school entry	Diph/Tet and oral polio vaccine or Diph/Tet/Polio vaccine.		These may be given, if desired, at 3 years of age to children entering nursery schools, attending day nurseries or living in children's homes.
Between 10 and 13 years of age	BCG vaccine		For tuberculin-negative children.
All girls aged 11 to 13 years	Rubella vaccine	There should be an interval of not less than 3 weeks between BCG and rubella vaccination.	All girls of this age should be offered rubella vaccine whether or not there is a past history of an attack of rubella.
At 15 to 19 years of age or on leaving school	Polio vaccine (oral or inactivated) and tetanus toxoid		

Rabies

Serious neurological complications in the form of demyelinating encephalomyelitis were recognised especially with the vaccine prepared in nerve tissue. Duck embryo vaccines and more modern vaccines derived from human diploid cells are safer.

Influenza

Severe generalised reactions almost akin to the attack of influenza itself may occur.

Whooping cough

Much controversy has surrounded the prophylaxis of whooping cough because of the possibilities of encephalopathy and convulsions, and an expert committee was set up by the Department of Health and Social Services in the United Kingdom recently to study all aspects of whooping cough and its prophylaxis. A report was published in 1977 and some of the conclusions are as follows:

1. Whooping cough remains a serious disease in young children and 10 per cent of those under two years of age have to be admitted to hospital.
2. Protective efficacy of the vaccine has been fully restored in recent years by changes in its antigens.
3. Many symptoms and signs purported to result from vaccination are not specific to pertussis vaccine, and retrospective analysis of cases of reported adverse reactions does not permit conditions such as childhood convulsions or encephalopathy that occur coincidentally and are unrelated to immunisation to be differentiated from those in which a relationship appears to exist.
4. A full course of immunisation with vaccine not only reduces the attack rate of the disease but also the severity of the illness.
5. Risks with current vaccines are slight, but care must be taken not to administer vaccines with a pertussis component where there are parental objections or medical contraindications such as pre-existing neurological conditions. (Diphtheria and tetanus components should still be given).
6. The first dose of triple vaccine should be given at three months of age so that more infants will be protected at the vulnerable period. Also at this earlier age there is a lower risk of febrile convulsions.

STERILISATION

Sterilisation is an absolute term and denotes the complete removal of all microorganisms from an object. There are several physical methods of sterilisation.

Heat

Dry heat and *moist heat* can be used.

Dry heat

This kills by causing oxidation of the bacterial cytoplasm and has the advantage of speed and of being easily controllable. Its use is restricted because certain articles, plastics, rubber goods and fabrics, cannot withstand high temperatures.

Simple flaming. This can be used for bacteriological loops and the points of forceps. Incineration is used for the disposal of contaminated carcasses, plastics and dressings.

Hot-air oven. This is a commonly used dry-heat steriliser. It is heated by electricity and has a fan to ensure even distribution of air. It is used for sterilising glassware, including glass syringes, powders, oils and greases that are impenetrable to moisture, as well as cotton wool pledgets and paraffin gauze dressings. Articles should be packed so as to allow circulation of the air. The *sterilisation time* is the sum of the *heat penetration time*, the *holding time*, the time required to sterilise a load when the required temperature has been reached, and the *safety time*, which is usually half the holding time. Glassware is generally sterilised by exposure to 160°C for one hour, or to 180°C for 20–30 minutes (the holding plus safety times) but these times may have to be doubled when powders, oils or greases are sterilised. The sterilisation cycle can take up to three hours including heat penetration and cooling times.

Conveyor oven. In a conveyor oven the method of sterilisation uses infra red radiation; the temperature of operation is 180°C for 10–15 minutes. This is used for large-scale sterilisation of glass syringes.

Moist heat

This kills by coagulation of the bacterial cytoplasm and is effective at lower temperatures than dry heat.

At temperatures below 100°C. *Pasteurisation* kills non-sporing pathogens. In the pasteurisation of milk two methods may be used: 64°–66°C for 30 minutes (the '*holder*' method), or 72°C for 15–20 seconds (the '*flash*' method). Vaccines are also inactivated at low temperatures such as 60°C for one hour.

At 100°C (boiling). Boiling at 100°C for five to ten minutes kills most vegetative organisms and some, but not all, spore-forming organisms;

it therefore does not ensure sterility. Boiling may be used for disinfecting contaminated crockery or cutlery.

At 100°C (steam). A temperature of 100°C is produced by pure steam in equilibrium with water boiling at normal atmospheric pressure and is used to sterilise substances such as bacteriological culture media that would be damaged by autoclaving. Steaming may be done either with a single exposure for 90 minutes, or with intermittent exposures, 20–30 minutes on three consecutive days (*Tyndallisation*). The principle underlying this practice is that the first steaming kills vegetative organisms and any spore-forming organisms present germinate before the next heating. These are then killed off during the next exposure to steam.

At temperatures above 100°C. The efficiency of steam under increased pressure as a *sterilising agent* is due to its condensation into a small volume of water when it meets the cooler surfaces of articles to be sterilised, liberating considerable latent heat to these surfaces. This is the principle involved in the *pressure cooker* and *autoclave*.

The autoclave

Two main groups of autoclaves are recognised; those used for porous loads such as dressings and preset operating theatre trays in hospitals, and those used as laboratory and instrument sterilisers.

The sterilisation cycle

This starts when the door of the autoclave is closed and ends with removal of the load and is as follows:

1. Removal of air from chamber
2. Sterilisation of the load
3. Exhaustion of steam from chamber after sterilisation
4. Drying and cooling of load

Removal of air from chamber

Air must be removed from the chamber for several reasons: (1) the presence of air seriously lowers the temperature at a given pressure; (2) air hinders the penetration of steam into porous materials such as surgical dressings; and (3) because air is denser than steam it forms a layer at the foot of the chamber of the autoclave and produces a lower temperature there.

Minimum exposure times for sterilisation of instruments are:

4 minutes at 133°C (at 30 lb/in^2)
15 minutes at 121°C (at 15 lb/in^2)
30 minutes at 115°C (at 10 lb/in^2)

Design of autoclaves

Design differences depend on the method of removing air from the chamber; there are two types in general use.

Downward displacement sterilisers. These are used in laboratories and as instrument sterilisers (Fig. 3.3). Steam enters near the top of the chamber and the air is displaced downwards through the load and the discharge channel at the bottom of the chamber. This channel is fitted with a thermostatic steam trap that remains open until all the air and condensate has been removed. Once pure steam only is present the temperature of the discharge rises to 121°C when the trap automatically closes and prevents further escape. Steam also enters the jacket independently and facilitates drying of the load. Once the sterilising cycle is completed the steam supply is stopped and filtered air enters the chamber to cool and dry the load.

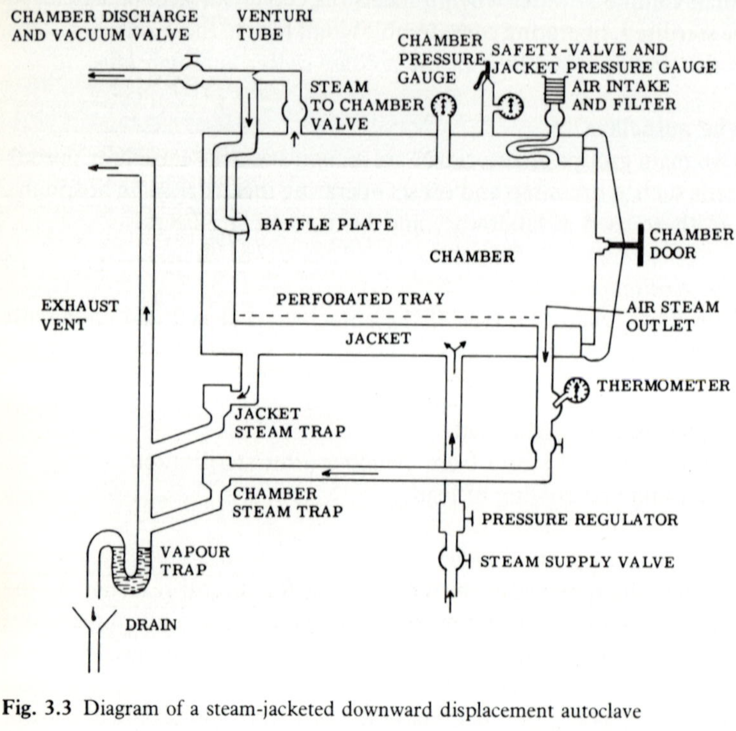

Fig. 3.3 Diagram of a steam-jacketed downward displacement autoclave

High pre-vacuum sterilisers. Used mostly in hospitals these are equipped with electrically-driven pumps that can remove virtually all the air from the chamber and this high vacuum ensures that steam penetrates the load rapidly. The effect of these sterilisers is to cut the sterilisation time; temperatures are higher (133°C) and pressures are greater (30 lb/in^2 gauge pressure). They are particularly useful when heat-sensitive materials have to be sterilised, because of the short sterilisation time.

Tests for efficiency of heat sterilisation

Chemical indicators
These are convenient because they give an immediate result, and may be placed inside or outside the load. Examples of such are *Browne's tubes*, small sealed tubes containing a red solution that turns to green when an adequate temperature has been maintained for a suitable time.

The Bowie-Dick autoclave tape test
This measures temperatures in packs and indicates the degree of steam penetration and air removal. A sheet of paper with a diagonal cross of autoclave tape is placed in a standard test pack, and a uniform colour change throughout the diagonal tape within a specified time indicates successful sterilisation.

Electrical indicators
Thermocouples are used to measure temperatures in loads in different areas of the steriliser. They are electrical leads that are connected to a recording instrument outside the steriliser which indicate the temperature reached during the autoclaving process.

Spore indicators
A preparation of bacterial spores such as *Bacillus stearothermophilus* is placed in a load and after autoclaving is tested for viability by transfer to another culture medium. It indicates the conditions of the load where it was placed but gives no indication of the sterilising performance in other loads.

Radiation
Two types of radiation are used, *non-ionising* and *ionising*.

1. *Non-ionising*. Bright sunlight can kill bacteria because of its ultraviolet rays. The effective rays are those with wavelengths of 24 000–28 000 nm (2400–2800 Å). Ultraviolet lamps emit rays within the above wavelengths but the value of these in sterilisation is very restricted because of their extremely poor penetrating power. They may be used for disinfection of work surfaces but spores are resistant to the rays.

2. *Ionising*. Ionising radiations are highly lethal. They may be either

high energy electrons (*cathode rays*) from a machine such as a linear accelerator or *gamma rays* from radioactive isotopes such as Cobalt 60. The mode of action of such radiations is to ionise vital cell components such as DNA, and a dose of 2.5 megarads (M rad) is generally adequate for this.

Articles that may be sterilised by radiation include disposable rubber gloves, needles and syringes, other plastic equipment and sutures. Advantages of this form of sterilisation are its efficiency, negligible rise in temperature and the fact that articles can be packed and sealed before sterilisation. Amongst the disadvantages are that textiles lose their tensile strength and colour, chemical changes occur in some products, and glassware darkens; in addition the sterilisation time is long.

Filtration

Various types of filter are used to remove organisms from fluids or from the air. Bacteria are trapped by direct impaction with the fibre or by electrostatic precipitation.

Fluids

Fluids and bacterial cultures can be rendered free from bacteria by using filters with a pore size of around 0.75 μm. Various types are used including *Chamberland* (unglazed porcelain), *Berkefeld* (diatomaceous earth) and *Seitz* (asbestos). Membrane filters of cellulose acetate and nitrate (*Millipore* and *Gradocol*) are available with specific pore sizes and are of particular use for filtering viruses.

Air

Air filtration is essential for operating theatres and isolation units; filters incorporate fibrous material such as glass wool, asbestos fibres in sheets, or gauze. Electrostatic precipitators are useful in trapping and removing particles from the air.

Gas

The most widely used gases are *ethylene oxide* and *formaldehyde*. They act by alkylating the –SH, –OH, –COOH or $-NH_2$ groups of proteins and nucleic acids under closely defined conditions of temperature and humidity. *Ethylene oxide* is used in hospitals and industrial processes but because of its explosive properties is unsuitable for fumigating rooms. It has a potent sporicidal action but is also toxic for man. It can diffuse easily through paper, plastics and fabrics and can be used for sterilising the following: swabs, electrical and dental equipment, components of the heart-lung machine, endoscopes, ureteric and cardiac catheters.

Formaldehyde
This gas is also highly lethal to organisms and spores and can be used in aqueous or gaseous forms. It is used for fumigating rooms and for disinfecting mattresses and bedding.

The advantages of sterilisation by gas lie in the fact that most articles are not damaged in the process and that penetration into porous materials is usually good.

DISINFECTION

Disinfection is not an absolute term like sterilisation, because although it implies destruction of bacteria it does not guarantee such an effect on spores or viruses.

Antisepsis. Antisepsis is the disinfection of living tissues and antiseptics are the milder disinfectants that can be allowed to come in contact with living tissue without causing harm.

Factors influencing the action of disinfectants

The action of disinfectants include protein and lipid denaturation in the cytoplasmic membrane, the blocking of biosynthetic pathways and damage to energy-yielding systems in the cell. Several factors influence their action:

Organisms
Most vegetative bacteria except acid-fast bacilli are killed under optimum conditions for disinfectant action, although spores and some viruses are highly resistant. Two per cent aqueous glutaraldehyde has proved effective against spores; viruses are also sensitive to this as well as to formaldehyde and iodine.

Rate of action
Some disinfectants act quickly, others slowly, depending on the number of organisms, whether they are protected by organic matter, the temperature and pH of the environment and the concentration of the disinfectant.

Number of organisms
In general the larger the numbers of organisms the longer the period of exposure required, and it should be remembered that bacteria may number many millions in situations where disinfectants are used.

Condition of organisms
Moisture in and around organisms is essential for disinfection.

Organic matter

Organic matter such as pus, blood and excreta, block penetration by coating the organisms; in addition, if there is much liquid organic matter this may serve to dilute and actually inactivate the disinfecting agents.

Concentration

The rate of killing of bacteria varies directly with the concentration of the disinfectant, and the failure of disinfection is often the result of failure to use recommended concentrations.

Temperature

A rise in temperature usually increases the rate of disinfection and disinfectants are more effective made up in hot water.

pH

This is important in the use of many disinfectants. An agent such as glutaraldehyde functions only in alkaline solutions, whereas compounds such as phenol work optimally in an acid medium.

Volume

Usually a greater volume of disinfectant produces more effective sterilisation as the effect of any inactivators present is reduced.

Formulation

Some disinfectants such as chlorhexidine operate best in an aqueous solution, or with 70 per cent alcohol. Some are combined with detergents in an attempt to achieve simultaneous disinfection and cleaning.

Deterioration

Many substances deteriorate when diluted with water and freshly-prepared solutions must be used. The longer the period the disinfectant is kept the less effective it will become, and bacteria have been known to survive and multiply in ageing disinfectants.

Inactivation

All disinfectants may be inactivated by certain materials. For example, hard water and soaps inactivate quaternary ammonium compounds and rubber inactivates phenols and chlorhexidine.

Evaluation of disinfectants

1. Manufacturers' tests

Disinfectants are frequently tested under conditions that may not be relevant to later *'in-use'* situations. Organic matter and inactivating materials may be absent, large volumes and high concentrations of the disinfectant may be used and the challenge may consist of only small numbers of bacteria. The *Rideal-Walker* test is a standard test and has been used for many years. It compares dilutions of the test disinfectant with known concentrations of phenol in the killing of *Salmonella typhi*. From the results a phenol coefficient is calculated; the higher the number the better the performance of the disinfectant. The calculation of the phenol coefficient is particularly *unhelpful* because (1) comparison with phenol has no meaning for any other type of disinfectant; (2) the conditions are not related to practical use (no organic matter is included for example); (3) only one species of organism is used; and (4) minor variations in technique can produce wide variations in the final result. Other phenol coefficient tests are the *AOAC* (Association of Official Agricultural Chemists) test which uses both *Salmonella typhi* and *Staphylococcus aureus*, and the *Chick-Martin* test which is a slight improvement in that it incorporates organic matter. It is only acceptable as a test for *phenolic* disinfectants however.

2. Reference laboratory tests
Tests carried out by the Disinfection Reference Laboratory of the Public Health Laboratory Service in London include the *Kelsey-Sykes* test which was introduced in 1969. It is suitable for all disinfectants and uses standard test strains of *Staphylococcus aureus*, *Pseudomonas aeruginosa*, *Proteus vulgaris* and *Escherichia coli*, grown on a chemically-defined medium; yeast cells are incorporated as a source of organic material.

3. In-use tests
Such tests assess the activity of a disinfectant in solutions that are actually in use in hospitals. They are much more realistic in that they take into account factors and circumstances that affect the performance of the disinfectant in a real-life situation.

CHEMICAL DISINFECTANTS

Alcohols

Examples
Isopropyl alcohol and ethyl alcohol.

Use
They are mainly used in 70 per cent concentrations diluted with water

and are useful as skin disinfectants before injections or venepuncture; they are also used for clean surfaces such as trolley tops.

Aldehydes

Examples
Formaldehyde
Glutaraldehyde

Use
Gaseous formaldehyde is used for fumigation: glutaraldehyde is useful for disinfection of clean instruments such as endoscopes but it is not suitable for use on dirty surfaces. It is irritant particularly to the eyes. Glutaraldehyde is also virucidal and is useful in situations where there may be a risk of serum hepatitis infection.

Diguanides

Examples
Chlorhexidine ('Hibitane')
Picloxidine

Use
Chlorhexidine is a useful disinfectant for skin and mucous membranes and is used as a 0.5 per cent concentration in 70 per cent alcohol. It is recommended as suitable for skin preparation of the patient, before sternal marrow aspiration, lumbar puncture and before surgery. It is not used for disinfection of instruments, equipment and surfaces because it is inactivated by many materials. 'Hibiscrub' (4 per cent chlorhexidine in detergent) is a useful preoperative scrub for surgeons' hands.

Halogens

Examples
Chlorine
Iodine
Iodophors: Povidone-iodine
'Betadine'
'Pevidine'
'Wescodyne'
Hypochlorites: 'Chloros'
'Milton'
'Domestos'
'Eusol'

Use

Chlorine is an effective disinfectant of water and *iodine* with alcohol is a powerful skin disinfectant which is recommended for use on patients before surgery. *Iodophors* contain iodine with surface active non-ionic detergents and are effective skin disinfectants because unlike iodine they do not stain or irritate the skin. They are sporicidal. *Hypochlorites*, derivatives of chlorine, are widely used for disinfecting dairy equipment and feeding bottles and are used in laboratory discard jars. Eusol is a solution of hypochlorites useful for wound cleansing. Hypochlorites are seriously inactivated by organic material, for example remains of milk in inadequately-cleaned feeding bottles and have a corrosive action on metals.

Phenolic compounds

Examples

Phenol (Carbolic acid)
Cresol
Chloroxylenol ('Dettol')
Clear soluble phenolic fluids: 'Lysol'
'Sudol'
'Hycolin'
White phenolic fluids ('Izal')
Black phenolic fluids ('Jeyes Fluid')
Hexachlorophane ('Phisohex')

Use

Phenolic compounds are widely-used disinfectants, although phenol itself is seldom if ever now used because of its irritant effect. The clear soluble fluids, white fluids and black fluids constitute *coal tar disinfectants* and are the basis of many proprietary disinfectants. They are widely used in disinfecting surfaces, in general sanitation and in laboratory discard jars. *Hexachlorophane* can be incorporated in detergents and soaps, and as 'Phisohex' is a useful skin disinfectant for a preoperative surgical scrub; it is retained on the skin for long periods and the antibacterial effect is slowly cumulative. There are possible hazards in using 'Phisohex' on infants as absorption with subsequent toxic effects may occur.

Quaternary ammonium compounds (QACs)

Examples

Cetrimide ('Cetavlon')
Benzalkonium chloride ('Roccal')

Cetrimide + chlorhexidine ('Savlon')
Cetrimide + picloxydine ('Resiguard')

Use
QACs are cationic detergents; the detergent effect on surface activity is due to an organic cation in solution. These *QACs* or *QACs + diguanides* have a powerful antibacterial activity and are widely used for wound and skin disinfection, for instrument disinfection and environmental sanitation.

Ampholytes

Example
'Tego' compounds

Use
These amphoteric compounds combine a detergent and bacteriocidal action and may be used in dairy and meat industries for environmental sanitation and application to surfaces.

SUMMARY OF MEDICAL APPLICATIONS OF CHEMICAL ANTISEPTICS AND DISINFECTANTS

Disinfection of skin

Mechanical removal of bacteria
A surgical scrub or shaving the patient's skin will reduce the skin flora but are not sufficient on their own. Chemical disinfection of the skin is essential although sterilisation is impossible. Desirable properties of skin disinfectants include rapidity and persistence of action with a bacteriocidal effect over a wide range of organisms; they should be non-irritant. Few agents meet these requirements.

Patient's skin

Before an injection
Soap and water
70 per cent ethyl or isopropyl alcohol with the addition of 1–2 per cent iodine or 0.5–1 per cent chlorhexidine.

Before surgery
Quaternary ammonium compounds (Cetrimide)
Alcoholic solution of iodine
Alcoholic solution of chlorhexidine
Chlorhexidine-cetrimide mixture ('Savlon')
Povidone-iodine solution

Surgeons' hands

Soap and water with a 'Savlon' or alcoholic chlorhexidine rinse.
Hexachlorophane surgical scrub
Povidone-iodine surgical scrub
'Hibiscrub'
These measures can also be used by nurses changing dressings.

Disinfection of clean, inanimate surfaces (trolleys, furniture)

Hypochlorite with detergent
70 per cent ethyl or isopropyl alcohol in water
0.1 per cent aqueous solution of chlorhexidine
0.1 per cent aqueous solution of cetrimide or benzalkonium chloride.

Disinfection of dirty surfaces (floors, toilets)

Phenolic compounds such as 'Lysol' and 'Sudol'

Disinfection of clean instruments and other apparatus

Buffered glutaraldehyde fluid
Ethylene oxide gas

FURTHER READING

Department of Health and Social Security (1977) *Whooping Cough Vaccination*. London: HMSO.

Lowbury, E. J. L., Ayliffe, G. A. J., Geddes, A. M. & Williams, J. D. (1975) *Control of Hospital Infection*. London: Chapman and Hall.

Maurer, I. M. (1974) *Hospital Hygiene*. London: Arnold.

Rubbo, S. D. and Gardner, J. F. (1965) *A Review of Sterilisation and Disinfection*. London: Lloyd-Luke.

Sykes, G. (1972) *Disinfection and Sterilisation*. London: Chapman and Hall.

Thompson, R. A. (1974) *The Practice of Clinical Immunology*. London: Arnold.

Weir, D. M. (1977) *Immunology. An Outline for Students of Medicine and Biology*. Edinburgh: Churchill Livingstone.

4

Diagnosis of infections

LIAISON WITH THE LABORATORY

Liaison between clinical and laboratory staff is of paramount importance in the investigation of a patient's illness and whenever there is the possibility of infection the bacteriologist, virologist or senior technician should be consulted about the laboratory investigations that should be undertaken. It is important for the clinician to give *relevant* information to the laboratory on the request form accompanying each specimen. Examples of information that may be important include the presentation of the patient's illness and the tentative clinical diagnosis; how long the person has been ill; whether he or she has been abroad recently; the relevant immunisation history and whether any antimicrobial therapy was given to the patient before the specimen was taken. For all specimens the date and hour of taking the specimen must be indicated.

The sooner a specimen reaches the laboratory the more reliable are the results that can be obtained and if specimens are important or urgent the doctor or nurse should deliver them personally. Swabs collected for virus isolation *must* be placed in a virological transport medium, and if a delay of more than two hours is anticipated they should be *refrigerated*.

Important and relevant laboratory findings will be reported immediately by most bacteriologists either in person or by telephone to the ward staff and before the typewritten report is despatched.

NOTES ON THE COLLECTION OF SPECIMENS

Swabs (see Fig. 4.1)

Numbers of organisms isolated from swabs in the laboratory may bear no relation to the numbers in the original clinical lesion. This is due to physical factors such as desiccation, to bacterial overgrowth and to the toxic effects of the metabolism of certain bacteria. In the laboratory

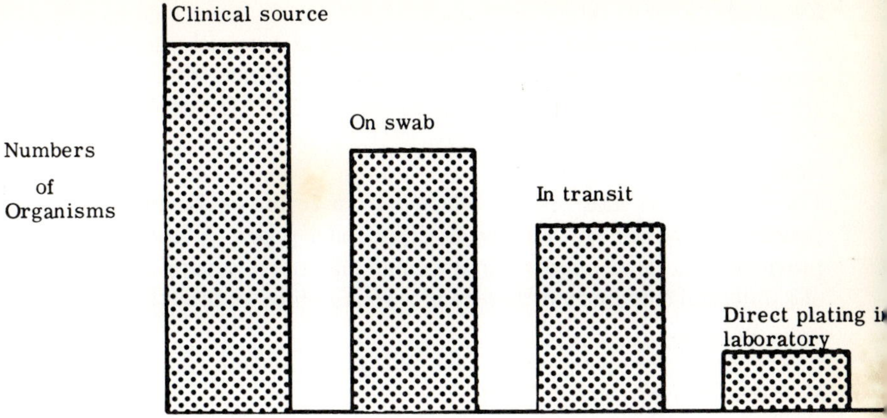

Fig. 4.1 Progressive loss of organisms from clinical source to laboratory

there is a loss of over 90 per cent of the organisms when swabs are plated out directly because many are retained on the swab. Transport media may be used in an attempt to maintain viability if the period of transit is to be long.

Blood for culture

Take blood before any chemotherapy, preferably 3–4 paired cultures per day at intervals. (Paired cultures are useful in checking for contaminants). Blood can be taken without waiting for a rigor. The site of venepuncture must be adequately cleansed (see Ch. 3). Use a bottle containing penicillinase if the patient is on penicillin or ampicillin. Most laboratories have an incubator available for blood cultures taken outwith laboratory hours. When blood is taken the needle should be changed before inoculating the broth medium; this will minimise the risk of contamination.

CSF

Place 2–3 ml in a sterile container. Contact the bacteriologist if meningitis is suspected.

Cervical swab

Take under direct vision (use a speculum) and in good light. In gonococcal infection plates are best inoculated at the bedside.

Cough plate (for whooping cough)

Plates are available from the laboratory on request. Expose to several coughs and return immediately to laboratory.

Eye swabs
Most causes of conjunctivitis are non-bacterial and special transport media for viruses and chlamydiae are available. Smears from swabs are best made in ward and dried in air; do not fix if for virology.

Faeces
The specimen is most easily collected from adults by having the patient pass faeces on to a wad of clean toilet paper. A 'spoon' is provided with the container. Send enough material to occupy a third of a universal container. A 'hot stool' is required for examination for cysts and ova.

Peritoneal dialysis fluids
Send in a dry sterile universal container.

Peritoneal, pericardial, pleural and joint fluids
Send in a special sterile bottle containing anticoagulant.

Pernasal swabs (for whooping cough)
Use a special, soft, wire-mounted swab. Pass it along the floor of the nasal cavity to the posterior wall of the naso-pharynx and rotate the swab gently.

Pus
Whenever possible aspirate pus and inflammatory exudates using a sterile syringe and needle. Send in sterile bijou or universal container.

Rectal swabs
These are inferior to a specimen of faeces.

Serological tests
5 ml of clotted blood should be despatched in a dry tube. 10 ml will be necessary if many tests are required. Paired samples are mandatory, an *acute phase* sample followed by a *convalescent phase* sample 10–14 days later. Fourfold rises in antibody titres are of diagnostic significance.

Smears
Best results are obtained if material is spread thinly on clean slides.

Sputum
Send as much sputum (*not* saliva) as possible in a sterile container. If tuberculosis is suspected and sputum is not obtainable consider gastric lavage or a laryngeal swab.

Surgical specimens
Send tissue in a dry sterile bottle. (There must be *no* fixative).

Urine
Catheter specimens (CSU). Collect urine directly from cathether, not the bag and do not allow the catheter to touch the container.

Midstream specimens (MSSU). To collect a *midstream* urine from females, the patient should be given the following instructions: (i) remove underclothing; (ii) wash the vulva and periurethral area with four separate sponges or swabs soaked in 10 per cent soft green soap solution, washing from the front backwards each time (green soap is preferred to water or saline, but disinfectant solutions must never be used); (iii) separate the labia majora with the fingers of one hand and, if necessary, prevent contamination from vaginal secretions by holding a swab between the labia minora; (iv) begin to pass urine into the toilet or bed-pan; (v) without interrupting the urine flow, collect the mid-portion of the stream in a wide-mouthed container (wax carton or glass 'honey-pot'); (vi) allow the terminal portion of the stream to pass into the toilet or bed-pan. The wide-mouthed container can be sealed and sent directly to the laboratory or urine can be transferred to a sterile disposable universal container.

An MSSU is easily collected from males.

Specimens from infants. Bag specimens are unsatisfactory. The child should be held over a container; an alternative is supra-pubic aspiration. In suspected tuberculosis at least 100 ml of early morning urine (first urine passed) (EMU) on three consecutive days should be collected.

Vaginal discharge
Vaginal swabs are taken when pyogenic infection or infection with *Candida* spp is suspected. Sponges should be used only for suspected *Trichomonas* infection. Cervical swabs are taken in uterine infection and in gonorrhoea.

INVESTIGATION OF INFECTIVE SYNDROMES

A general approach must be adopted in assessing the microbial aetiology of infections because of the possible involvement of organisms other than bacteria.

Protocols of investigation

Pyrexia of uncertain origin
This can be defined as a fever, constant or intermittent, with no

immediately obvious cause, lasting for at least four days. Frequent blood cultures should be taken, 3–4 per day, until the diagnosis is made, and serum samples should be provided for estimations of antibodies to *Brucella*, *Leptospira*, *Toxoplasma*, *Mycoplasma pneumoniae*, *Coxiella burneti* (Q fever), *Chlamydia* and viruses such as adenovirus, influenza virus, cytomegalovirus, mumps, measles and Varicella-zoster. Deep sepsis, endocarditis, tuberculosis and exotic protozoal and fungal infections should be considered in the differential diagnosis.

Send faeces and urine for culture of *Salmonella*.

Actinomycosis
Analysis of specimens of pus is preferable to processing swabs (a general principle).

Adenopathy, adenitis
Brucellosis and tuberculosis should be considered and serological tests should be performed for infectious mononucleosis (Paul-Bunnell) and other virus infections.

Anthrax
In the United Kingdom *malignant pustule* is the commonest presentation. Take swabs from the lesion.

Arthritis
Aspirate joint effusion for culture; paired sera to check for rubella and hepatitis B should be obtained.

Brucellosis
Repeated blood cultures in special medium (*Castaneda*) are the most useful investigations, in addition to serum for agglutinating and complement-fixing antibodies.

Conjunctivitis
Smears should be made and material for bacterial culture should be plated out at the bedside.

Causative organisms are often non-bacterial, such as *Chlamydia*, (Trachoma-inclusion conjunctivitis) *Herpes simplex*, adenovirus and *Molluscum contagiosum*.

Deep sepsis
Blood culture is useful if the aetiological agent is from inaccessible or unlocated sites.

Diarrhoea

Non-infectious causes should be considered. Infectious causes include *Salmonella, Shigella, Campylobacter*, enteropathogenic *Escherichia coli* in infants, food-poisoning organisms, vibrios, viruses and amoebae. Repeated stool specimens and blood cultures are required.

Endocarditis

At least 3–4 blood cultures per day for several days are necessary. If cultures are consistently negative Q fever or psittacosis should be considered and a check should be made to ensure that the patient is not receiving antibiotics. (This should be done in any situation where there are unexpected negative findings).

Food-poisoning

Salmonella spp, for example *typhimurium* and *newport, Staphylococcus aureus, Clostridium welchii, Bacillus cereus, Vibrio parahaemolyticus* or *Campylobacter* spp are the most likely bacterial causes. Stool specimens and any samples of suspected foodstuffs should be sent for examination.

Gangrene

Blood cultures and specimens of pus and necrotic tissues are optimal specimens.

Gonoccoccal infection

Smears should be made and cultures taken from all relevant sites; cervix, urethra, rectum, throat and conjunctiva using Thayer-Martin medium or New York City medium. Vaginal swabs are of little use. The Gonococcal complement-fixation test (GCFT) is not reliable.

Hepatitis

Blood is required for hepatitis B (Australia) antigens and antibody tests and paired sera for antibodies to Epstein-Barr virus, *Herpes simplex* virus and *Cytomegalovirus*.

Leptospirosis

Blood culture in special media and serological studies are indicated.

Meningitis

Cerebrospinal fluid (CSF) and blood cultures are needed for bacteriology and CSF and faeces for virology.

Osteomyelitis
Blood cultures are essential. Pus should be sent for culture.

Pneumonia
Sputum, for culture of bacterial and fungal pathogens, throat washings and paired sera for *Mycoplasma pneumoniae, Psittacosis,* Q fever and influenza virus, will cover the range of investigations required for the most likely aetiological agents.

Puerperal pyrexia
Blood, cervical swabs and urine specimens should be cultured.

Septicaemia
Frequent blood cultures are required in addition to screening for underlying causes.

Sore throat
A throat swab and specimen of saliva should be examined; if these are negative take serum for a Paul-Bunnell test.

Syphilis
10 ml clotted blood are required for screening tests, for example *Treponema pallidum* haemagglutination test (TPHA), and the Venereal Diseases Research Laboratory test (VDRL). Other tests such as the Reiter protein complement fixation test (RPCF) and fluorescent-antibody tests may be available.

Urinary tract infection
Urine (CSU or MSU) should be despatched quickly to laboratory or refrigerated if a delay of more than 4 hours is expected.

Vaginal discharge
Swabs will be examined for *Candida* and pyogenic infection and exudate (sponge) for Trichomonads.

DIAGNOSTIC APPROACHES IN BACTERIOLOGY

The objects of diagnostic bacteriology are two-fold; firstly, to identify the causative organisms of infection in the patient and, secondly, to establish whether the results of infection, namely antibodies, are present in the patient's serum. Before a specific organism can be accepted as the cause of a specific infection certain criteria, known as the *KOCH-HENLE* postulates, must be satisfied. These state that the organism must be present in the host and be able to be isolated in pure culture from the infected lesions; that the infection can be reproduced when the organisms from the pure culture are inoculated into a susceptible species; and that the organisms can be re-isolated during the course of the experimental disease. These postulates are now supplemented by demonstration of an increase in the antibody titre to the infecting organisms during the course of the disease.

Laboratory methods of diagnosis

Inspection

A specimen should be carefully inspected with the naked eye for any features that may be diagnostically significant, such as pus and mucus in the stool of a case of bacillary dysentery and 'sulphur granules' in the pus of a case of actinomycosis. It is also important to ensure that the specimen indicated on the request form is the one that arrives in the laboratory and that it has been properly taken; that a specimen of sputum is not a specimen of saliva, that a specimen of tissue is not in fixative and that a rectal swab does not appear lily-white.

Microscopy

Direct wet films are important in the examination of faeces for cysts and parasites and vaginal exudates for trichomonads. Fixed films are routinely made in the examination of sputum, urine and wound swabs and are commonly stained by Gram's method; they reveal the presence of pus cells, red blood cells and organisms. Other stains can be used such as the Ziehl-Neelsen for tubercle bacilli, Albert's for corynebacteria and methyl violet for Vincent's organisms. In the examination of skin lesions, faeces and throat swabs the Gram film may not be helpful although it can indicate the appropriate method of culture. Only very occasionally can it be reasonably diagnostic, as in the demonstration of Vincent's organisms from a mouth swab or gingival scrapings and Gram-negative intracellular diplococci from the cerebrospinal fluid of a case of meningitis.

Phase contrast microscopy is useful in the investigation of spirochaetal infections and *fluorescent antibody techniques* are of value in the direct demonstration of organisms in clinical material, namely *Bordetella pertussis* in nasopharyngeal swabs, *Treponema pallidum* in exudates and *Neisseria gonorrhoeae* in urethral discharge.

Culture

Culture is essential in the diagnostic process and the specimen may have to be processed before culture; for example, sputum is homogenised, many fluids are centrifuged and the deposit cultured. Blood agar is a commonly used medium in medical bacteriology, but many others are available, including *selective media*; these incorporate substances that prevent the growth of certain species but allow the growth of others. The addition of crystal violet to blood agar may be useful in the diagnosis of skin infection as it inhibits staphylococci but permits the growth of *Streptococcus pyogenes*. Similarly, the addition of potassium tellurite makes the isolation of corynebacteria from a throat swab more possible by inhibiting growth of many of the throat commensals. Nalidixic acid and sodium azide can be added to culture media to inhibit Gram-negative bacilli, and the incorporation of certain aminoglycosides such as gentamicin and neomycin in culture media facilitates growth of clostridia and beta-haemolytic streptococci by inhibiting growth of commensal flora.

Blood agar plates may be incubated aerobically or anaerobically and frequently both methods are used. Culture plates can be incubated anaerobically in an anaerobic cabinet or in an anaerobic jar from which oxygen has been removed and replaced either by hydrogen or a hydrogen-carbon dioxide mixture from a gas cylinder. Commercially-produced envelopes are available which produce anaerobic conditions within the jars when water is added. Liquid media such as Robertson's meat broth also produce anaerobic conditions in the meat particles at the bottom of the tubes. Finally, many cultures grow better in an atmosphere of 5–10 per cent carbon dioxide, for example gonococci, and many laboratories now use incubation in carbon dioxide for routine specimens.

Biochemical tests

Many bacteria have a characteristic biochemical profile which may be of value in their identification. A great many of these are known, including:

Enzyme production

A few examples are coagulase from *Staphylococcus aureus*, lecithinase from *Clostridium welchii* and oxidase from *Neisseria gonorrhoeae*.

Sugar fermentation tests

These are useful in the identification of the enterobacteriaceae. Various sugars are used and are checked for the production of acid, gas or both by the bacteria.

Serological tests

These are of two different forms, *direct* for detection of antigen and *indirect* for detection of antibody.

Detection of antigen. Agglutination tests on slides and in tubes and precipitation methods in capillary tubes and agar gel are available. Living suspensions of the unknown organisms are used and these are tested against a range of antisera of known identity. Fluorescent antibody and coagglutination tests for certain antigens may also be performed.

In recent years *counterimmunoelectrophoresis* (*CIE*) has been used in the detection of many antigens, such as those present in meningococci, pneumococci, streptococci, salmonellae, *Haemophilus influenzae* and *Proteus* spp.

Detection of antibody. Various tests are used when it is not possible to isolate the organism from the patient's tissues. By demonstrating serum antibodies to suspected organisms it is inferred that the patient is infected with the organism. A single test is totally inadequate because if the antibody titre is raised it is impossible to say whether this is due to past or present infection. Two tests must be done, one at the beginning of the illness and the other 10–14 days later, and if a rising titre or level of antibodies is demonstrated between the two specimens (ideally a fourfold difference) it can be said that the patient's infection is current. It is usual to test for *agglutinating* and *complement-fixing* antibodies which are highly specific, as for example in the serological diagnosis of brucellosis. Other tests that have proved of value for detection of antibody in more recent times are *radioimmunoassay* (*RIA*) which is specific, sensitive and requires only small quantities of antigen, and *enzyme-linked immunosorbent-assay* (*ELISA*) which has been successfully used to detect antibodies against streptococci, salmonellae, cholera vibrios and *Treponema pallidum*. Non-specific tests are also available, including the *Paul-Bunnell* test for infectious mononucleosis and the *Wassermann Reaction* for syphilis. Tests can also be done on the patient, for example the *Schick test* which demonstrates antitoxic immunity to diphtheria and the *tuberculin test* which tests for previous contact with *Mycobacterium tuberculosis*.

Special tests applied to isolates

These include epidemiological markers such as bacteriophage typing for staphylococci, colicine production by *Shigella sonnei* and pyocine production by *Pseudomonas aeruginosa*.

Animal tests

In bacteriology these are used to test whether organisms such as clostridia and corynebacteria are toxigenic and in the diagnosis of tuberculosis. They may be useful in virology, for example in the isolation of Coxsackie group A viruses by intraperitoneal inoculation of suckling mice.

Antibiograms

The laboratory identification of organisms is incomplete without determining their antibiotic sensitivity patterns. Different strains of the same bacterial species may be identified by their different antibiograms.

Interpretation of laboratory findings

Interpretation of findings is not always an easy matter. In some instances it can be relatively simple as, for example, the isolation of *Staphylococcus aureus* from a septic skin lesion, or *Mycobacterium tuberculosis* from the sputum of a patient with respiratory symptoms. On the other hand the isolation of *Neisseria meningitidis* from the throat of a patient with meningitis, or *Streptococcus pyogenes* from the throat of a patient complaining of sore throat may merely indicate simple carriage of these organisms; viruses may have been the causes of infection in both cases. A single isolation of *Staphylococcus aureus* from the blood of a patient with suspected infective endocarditis may not be of diagnostic significance but repeated isolations of the organisms of the same phage type confirm the diagnosis. Knowledge of the normal flora of the various areas of the body can frequently resolve the problem of identifying which organisms are contaminants, and information as to the approximate numbers of organisms in a specimen is helpful because contaminants are frequently present in smaller numbers than the organism causing the disease. Antibody tests can also be used for clarification of the cause. The response to antibiotics chosen on the basis of antibiograms of the organisms presumed to be the cause may be helpful. For example, failure of response to penicillin in a patient with pneumonia and penicillin-sensitive pneumococci should raise the suspicion that some other agent such as penicillin-resistant *Staphylococcus aureus* may be responsible.

Increasingly the role of endogenous organisms in infections is being realised and this makes valid interpretation of laboratory findings difficult. In this complex area close clinical and laboratory collaboration is essential.

FURTHER READING

Cruickshank, R., Duguid, J. P., Marmion, B. P. & Swain, R. H. A. (1973) *Medical Microbiology*. Edinburgh: Churchill Livingstone.

Passmore, R. & Robson, J. S. (1973) *A Companion to Medical Studies*. Oxford: Blackwell Scientific Publications.

Rytel, M. W. (1975) Rapid diagnostic methods in infectious diseases. *Advances in Internal Medicine*, **20**, 37–60.

Stokes, E. J. (1975) *Clinical Bacteriology*. London: Arnold.

5

Treatment of infections

ANTIBIOTICS AND CHEMOTHERAPY

Principles of use

Is an antibiotic necessary?
Antibiotics are often administered totally unnecessarily. In the author's experience they have been given for the common cold, flea bites, sebaceous cysts, a sprained ankle and bleeding from the urinary tract. Antibiotics, frequently prescribed for such lesions as a superficial collection of pus cannot penetrate formed pus, nor can they penetrate adequately fibrin and granulation tissue. Usually simple surgical drainage is all that is required. In deciding whether or not to use an antibiotic toxicity reactions and side effects must be kept in mind and although some antimicrobial agents produce more serious side effects than others none is absolutely safe. Even penicillin which is accepted as one of the safer antibiotics can produce serious and sometimes fatal hypersensitivity reactions in a few people. The advantages and disadvantages of antibiotic therapy must be weighed up carefully for each invidual.

The choice of drug
This depends primarily on the nature of the infecting organism and its antibiotic sensitivity pattern. Antibiotics should be used on a rational bacteriological basis although there is a place for an *educated guess* in a clinical emergency such as septicaemia, or osteomyelitis in a child. Consideration must be given as to whether a bacteriocidal or bacteriostatic drug of broad or narrow spectrum should be used.

Bacteriocidal and bacteriostatic action. Antimicrobial drugs may be bacteriocidal and rapidly kill bacteria, or bacteriostatic and inhibit multiplication without actually killing the organisms. The line of demarcation between the two actions is not clear cut and is dependent on factors such as the extent of the bacterial challenge, the concentration of the drug and the organism concerned; some drugs such as erythromycin are bacteriostatic at normal dosage but are bacteriocidal in higher concentrations. Theoretically bacteriocidal drugs are to be preferred to bacteriostatic drugs; however, a critical factor in the cure of infection is the patient's own defence system and bacteriostatic drugs may be able to inhibit multiplication of the bacteria sufficiently to allow their elimination by the white cells.

Broad-spectrum and narrow-spectrum drugs. Antimicrobial drugs differ in the range of bacteria they inhibit. Broad-spectrum drugs such as the tetracyclines and ampicillin have a wide range of activity against both Gram-positive and Gram-negative bacteria, whereas flucloxacillin has a narrow spectrum. It is very effective against *Staphylococcus aureus* but ineffective against almost all Gram-negative bacteria. Narrow-spectrum drugs are to be preferred because of their greater specificity and unlike broad-spectrum drugs they do not have the same adverse effects on the normal flora of the body. Broad-spectrum drugs can so alter the composition of the flora at various sites that its normal protective effect is ruined, and it is well recognised that certain pathogenic organisms can colonise such areas and produce superinfection, as in infection of the mouth by *Candida* spp.

Combinations of drugs

In general a single antimicrobial drug should be used for the treatment of a particular infection but there are indications for the use of a combination of drugs. These are: (1) to achieve a synergistic effect, the combination of drugs producing a much greater effect than either drug alone; (2) to prevent the development of bacterial resistance; (3) to deal with mixed infections.

In the treatment of infective endocarditis caused by *Streptococcus faecalis* it has been shown that a combination of a penicillin and an aminoglycoside is often therapeutic whereas this would not be so with full doses of either drug alone. Synergism is well demonstrated in the laboratory in the combination of sulphonamide and trimethoprim in the drug *cotrimoxazole*. The use of combinations of drugs to prevent the emergence of drug-resistant strains is well demonstrated in the treatment of tuberculosis. In this disease treatment is prolonged and resistance to single drugs occurs quickly. The incidence of mutants resistant to a single drug may be in the order of $1:10^7$ cell divisions so that if two drugs are given the chances are then only $1:10^{14}$.

Combinations of drugs should not be used either empirically in mixed infections or when the diagnosis is obscure, although an important exception is when a person is seriously ill and no bacteria have been isolated. Some combinations theoretically may be *antagonistic*; for example, penicillin acts on organisms that are actively growing and if it is combined with a bacteriostatic drug this action may be prevented.

Fixed-dosage preparations (commercial preparations) must be used with caution, because the proportion of each drug may be wrong for the particular infection to be treated and there is no scope for altering these proportions.

General considerations

Antibiotics should be given in therapeutic doses, for an adequate period. If after a few days' treatment there is no clinical response it usually means either that the infecting organisms are resistant, in which case further specimens should be sent to the laboratory, or that the drug is failing to reach the bacteria in sufficient concentration. *Local treatment* should be carried out with antibiotics such as neomycin that are not used systemically, because if drug resistance occurs a valuable systemic drug becomes useless for treatment of serious infection in that patient. *Side effects* of drugs should be known and the drug of choice should be the one that incorporates minimal side effects with maximum efficiency, although this is not always possible with organisms that are multiply-resistant. *Drug incompatibility* must be remembered. Nalidixic acid, for example, potentiates the action of warfarin and severe bleeding may ensue.

Prophylactic use of drugs

Surveys conducted on aspects of prophylaxis have frequently reported that an increase in resistance to the antibiotics used can occur and that widespread prophylactic use may predispose to infections with more resistant organisms by altering the composition of the protective commensal flora or by selecting out resistant mutants. Ironically a substantial number of reports have stated that patients on prophylactic drugs, particularly those undergoing surgery, have a higher infection rate than those in non-treated control groups because the antibiotics prescribed are frequently totally inappropriate for the bacteria that subsequently cause the infections.

There are however some clear and justifiable indications for prophylaxis. In trauma, when there are the possibilities of tetanus or gas gangrene if the wound becomes contaminated by *Clostridium tetani* or *Clostridium welchii*, benzyl or phenoxymethyl penicillin should be given. Following thigh amputation in the elderly there is a risk of endogenous infection from *Clostridium welchii* and a similar policy should be followed. Children who have had a primary attack of rheumatic fever run a high risk of a subsequent attack and phenoxymethyl penicillin should be given to them to prevent reinfection with *Streptococcus pyogenes*. Antibiotics have proved useful in the prevention of infective endocarditis in those with damaged valves, valve prostheses or congenital malformations, when undergoing dental extraction.

Within these widely different sets of circumstances there are grey areas where there can be arguments for or against prophylaxis, as in open heart surgery and before anaesthesia in patients with chronic respiratory disease.

It should be recognised that the inherent dangers of the prophylactic use of antibiotics may far outweigh the mental balm and sense of security produced by the use of the prophylactic agent.

Mode of action of antimicrobial agents

There are five main modes of action of antibiotics:

Inhibition of cell-wall synthesis

Drugs that prevent cell-wall synthesis do so by inhibiting the transpeptidase step required for cross-linking the polysaccharide chains in the peptidoglycan layer of the cell wall. The *penicillins*; *cephalosporins* and *cycloserine* act in this way.

Damage to cell membrane

Some antibiotics produce damage by binding to the membrane, acting as cationic detergents, resulting in the loss of the semipermeable properties of the membrane. Substances then pass out from the cell and death occurs. Polypeptide antibiotics such as *polymyxin* act in this fashion.

Inhibition of protein synthesis

Antibiotics causing this have an effect on *translation* in the cell and include *chloramphenicol*; the *tetracyclines*; the *aminoglycosides* such as *streptomycin, neomycin, kanamycin* and *gentamicin*; *erythromycin*; *lincomycin* and *clindamycin*.

Inhibition of nucleic acid synthesis

Nalidixic acid inhibits replication of DNA and rifampicin blocks transcription in prokaryotic cells.

Inhibition of folate synthesis

Sulphonamides and *trimethoprim* block different steps in folate synthesis in bacteria. Folic acid is needed as a cofactor in the synthesis of thymidine and other nucleotides.

Resistance of bacteria to antimicrobial drugs

Bacteria may be *naturally* resistant to a particular antibiotic but they may also *acquire* resistance to drugs. The two mechanisms whereby bacteria initially sensitive to an antibiotic may become resistant are by *mutation* and *gene transfer*.

Mutation

Mutations develop spontaneously in bacterial cultures at a frequency of one per 10^7–10^9 cell divisions, whether or not a drug has been administered. The resistant mutants that occur in the presence of antibiotic are not as robust as the parent strains and do not survive for long if the drug is discontinued. If, however, there is continued exposure to the antibiotic, sensitive parent strains will be killed whereas the resistant mutants will remain viable and multiply. The action of the drug therefore is to *select* the resistant bacteria.

The mechanism of resistance depends on the mode of action of the drug. For example, mutations may produce decreased affinity of the target site or reduced penetration of the drug into the cell.

Gene transfer

This can occur by *transduction* or *conjugation* and consists of transfer of genetic material from a strain or species previously resistant to one or more antibiotic to a strain previously sensitive. In these cases genes for drug resistance are carried on extrachromosomal elements or *plasmids*.

Transduction

Penicillin resistance in *Staphylococcus aureus* depends on the presence of a plasmid carrying the gene for penicillinase (beta-lactamase) production. These plasmids can be transferred amongst different staphylococcal strains by bacteriophages.

Conjugation

R-factors (plasmids bearing drug-resistance genes) may be spread by conjugation amongst cells of a wide range of species, notably the *enterobacteria* and *Pseudomonas aeruginosa*. Contact between donor and recipient cells is required and the genetic material is transferred directly between the two cells.

Selection

Selection by antibiotics is important whether resistance is produced by mutation or gene transfer. Repeated exposure of bacteria to the drug together with long periods of exposure in the population means that more resistant strains will be selected out. An important step in limiting the increasing number of resistant strains is to reduce the use of the drug. This should allow the return of the sensitive strains.

Laboratory control of antibiotic therapy

Such assays include tests on the organism as well as measurement of responses in the patient.

Tests on the organism

These are essentially of two types, *dilution tests* and *disk sensitivity tests*.

Tube dilution tests. These methods are too time-consuming for routine use but they are carried out from time to time in all laboratories. They indicate the minimum inhibitory concentration (MIC) of a drug required for a specific organism in various diseases, such as infective endocarditis, thereby ensuring a more accurate and effective dose regimen. The MIC is read from the tube containing the highest dilution of the antibiotic to inhibit growth.

Agar plate dilution tests. These are useful when a large number of strains have to be tested. Various dilutions of the antibiotic are prepared in agar plates and each plate is seeded with several strains. After incubation the MIC of the drug can be readily ascertained from the plate that contains the highest dilution of the antibiotic required to prevent growth of the test strain.

Disk diffusion tests. These are inherently less accurate than dilution tests but are more rapid and convenient. Disks are made of filter paper impregnated with a known amount of antibiotic and placed on an agar plate that has been inoculated with the test organism. After incubation the plate is examined for zones of inhibition around the disks where the antibiotic has diffused into the medium. Standardisation of results is important in such tests and this can be done in one of two ways: (1) correlation of the diameter of the zone with a scale relating zone size to the MIC. Examples are the Ericsson and Kirby-Bauer methods; (2) the zone size produced by the organism is compared with the zone size given by a control organism tested by the same method. Many variables can affect the results of such tests, such as inoculum size, composition of the medium, antibiotic content of the disk and pH, but the main advantage of such tests is that the clinician can be informed of the results in the shortest possible time.

Tests of responses in the patient

Assays can be done on the serum, urine, sputum or cerebrospinal fluid and these measure whether effective concentrations of an antibiotic are being attained. They are also useful in guarding against excessively high serum levels of antibiotics with serious side effects. *Tube dilutions* and *agar diffusion* methods may be used.

In *tube dilutions,* graded dilutions of the fluid to be tested, usually serum, are made in a liquid medium; a standard inoculum of bacteria of known sensitivity, usually NCTC strains, for example *Staphylococcus aureus,* NCTC 6571, the *Oxford* staphylococcus, is then added. After incubation the tubes are examined for turbidity and the tube that contains the highest dilution of serum to inhibit growth of the organisms is noted. The MIC of the Oxford staphylococcus is known for each antibiotic and this allows calculation of the amount of antibiotic present in the patient's undiluted serum. It can also be helpful to check the patient's serum levels of antibiotic against the organism isolated.

Agar diffusion methods. In these holes are cut in the agar previously inoculated with a control organism. The holes are filled with the serum under test and zones of inhibition produced by the antibiotic in the serum are compared with a graph of the sizes of zones produced by known concentrations of the antibiotic.

In guarding against excessive serum levels of a potentially toxic antibiotic, estimations can be made by testing serum taken about one hour after a dose (*peak level*) and serum taken just before the next dose (*trough level*). *Rapid assays* may from time to time be required particularly in monitoring treatment with aminoglycosides during renal failure when results may be needed on the same day. Rapid plate assays are available and other methods include a *urease assay, radio-immune assays, radio-tagging assays* and an *immunofluorescence polarisation assay.*

ANTIMICROBIAL DRUGS OF CLINICAL IMPORTANCE

Sulphonamides

Antibacterial spectrum and uses

These drugs have a broad-spectrum, bacteriostatic effect. They are effective against certain Gram-positive organisms such as pneumococci but their use against these organisms has been superseded by other drugs. Some Gram-negative cocci are sensitive and likewise many enterobacteria. Sulphonamides are used against Gram-negative bacilli, for example in urinary tract infection caused by *Escherichia coli*; certain non-absorbable varieties can be used for preoperative preparation of the bowel.

Mode of action

Sulphonamides are structural analogues of para-aminobenzoic acid (PABA) which is involved in the synthesis of folic acid by bacteria. They inhibit bacterial growth by competitive inhibition of the enzymes involved in the incorporation of PABA into the folate pathway. Humans cannot synthesise folates and have to absorb them from the intestine, thus sulphonamides show selective toxicity by inhibiting a synthetic pathway not present in the host's cells.

Resistance

Many species, particularly meningococci, in the past sensitive to the sulphonamides, are now resistant and this applies also to other bacteria. Resistance can be produced by synthesis of a folic acid synthetase that has a lowered affinity for sulphonamide, or by over-production of PABA. Cross resistance in the group is complete.

Cotrimoxazole

Antibacterial spectrum and uses

Cotrimoxazole is a combination of a *sulphonamide* (sulphamethoxazole) and *trimethoprim* and has a bacteriocidal action. Although it is effective against certain Gram-positive species and *Haemophilus influenzae* cotrimoxazole is particularly useful against many of the enterobacteria that cause *urinary tract infection.* It can also be used in typhoid fever and brucellosis.

Mode of action

Trimethoprim is a synthetic agent that in concert with sulphonamides produces a sequential blockade of folic acid synthesis in bacteria. The combination produces a strongly-synergistic action and the effect of the combination is equal to about ten times the effect of trimethoprim alone.

Resistance

Although this can be produced easily in the laboratory by the transmission of R-factors it is not yet a problem clinically.

The penicillins

The following will be considered: *Benzyl penicillin, phenoxymethyl, cloxacillins, ampicillin* (*amoxycillin, talampicillin*), *carbenicillin* and *carfecillin.*

Mode of action (all penicillins)

Penicillins act by inhibiting the transpeptidase step required for cross-linking the polysaccharide chains in the peptidoglycan layer of the cell wall. All are bacteriocidal.

Benzyl penicillin (penicillin G)

This was the original penicillin and is still the most effective against *Streptococcus pyogenes* and non-penicillinase producing *Staphylococcus aureus*, pneumococci, clostridia and many neisseriae. It is useful against *Bacillus anthracis* and *Actinomyces israelii* but Gram-negative bacilli such as the enterobacteria and *Pseudomonas* spp are highly resistant to it. It is inactivated by gastric acid and has to be given parenterally.

Resistance. Many strains of *Staphylococcus aureus* are now resistant because of the production of a penicillin-destroying enzyme (beta-lactamase) that hydrolyses the beta-lactam ring in the penicillin nucleus. Such strains are much more common in hospital and are spread by cross infection and selected out by continued use of the drug. In the community there is increasing resistance to penicillin in gonococci due either to mutation or the production of a beta-lactamase obtained via R-factors from *Escherichia coli.* Some Gram-negative bacilli produce beta-lactamases and this makes them resistant to benzyl penicillin and also to other penicillins such as ampicillin.

Phenoxymethyl penicillin (penicillin V)

Antibacterial spectrum and uses. This drug can be given orally because it is acid stable and it has much the same antibacterial spectrum as benzyl penicillin, although in serious systemic infection it is preferable to give high doses of benzyl penicillin. Phenoxyethyl and phenoxypropyl penicillins exist but none is better than phenoxymethyl.

Resistance. This is the same as for benzyl penicillin.

Cloxacillins

Antibacterial spectrum and uses. These belong to the group of semi-synthetic penicillins that are produced by chemical manipulation of the penicillin nucleus. *Methicillin* was the first of this group to be introduced, then *cloxacillin* and *flucloxacillin*. *Methicillin* has now been largely superseded as it has to be given by injection because of its instability in gastric juice. *Cloxacillin* can be given orally or parenterally; *flucloxacillin* is a pharmacological improvement on cloxacillin. These penicillins are used against penicillinase-producing staphylococci because their penicillin molecule is not affected by penicillinase. For infections caused by penicillin-sensitive organisms they are less effective than benzyl or phenoxymethyl penicillins.

Resistance. Resistance, though uncommon, does occur clinically; this is not due to production of a beta-lactamase, but probably to mutation.

Ampicillin

Antibacterial spectrum and uses. This semi-synthetic penicillin has a far wider spectrum of activity than the other pencillins and is a *broad-spectrum antibiotic.* It is destroyed by penicillinase and is therefore of no value against the penicillinase-producing *Staphylococcus aureus.* In general, it is much less active than benzyl penicillin against most Gram-positive cocci and should not be used for infections with such organisms, although an exception is infection caused by *Streptococcus faecalis.* It is effective against many Gram-negative organisms such as *Escherichia coli* (although resistance is increasing), *Haemophilus influenzae,* non-penicillinase-producing *Proteus* spp *Shigella* and *Salmonella.*

Resistance. Many enterobacteria are now resistant due to R-factor beta-lactamase production.

Amoxycillin

The antibacterial activity is similar to ampicillin but amoxycillin is better absorbed producing higher serum levels.

Talampicillin

This is an inactive compound that is hydrolysed in the intestine to form ampicillin. Dose for dose it produces higher serum levels than ampicillin.

Carbenicillin

Antibacterial spectrum and uses. This is a semi-synthetic penicillin that has a special use in treatment of infections caused by *Pseudomonas aeruginosa* in particular, and some *Proteus* infections, as well as other enterobacteria. It is not effective against Gram-positive organisms.

Resistance. Carbenicillin is inactivated by penicillinase.

Carfecillin

This is the phenyl ester of carbenicillin and has the advantage of increased absorption from the intestine.

The cephalosporins

Antibacterial spectrum and uses

The cephalosporin family of antibiotics is related to the penicillins. Many semi-synthetic derivatives are available with different properties, but the available compounds do not show such marked differences in their antibacterial spectrum as in the penicillin family. *Cephaloridine* and *cephalothin* are given parenterally and *cephalexin* orally. All have a broad spectrum of activity inhibiting both Gram-positive cocci and Gram-negative bacilli, but most infections are more effectively treated with the appropriate penicillin unless the patient is hypersensitive to penicillin. This would seem to be the main indication for using cephalosporins, although cross hypersensitivity may occur.

Mode of action

Cephalosporins are bacteriocidal, acting on the growing cell wall in a similar manner to the penicillins.

Resistance

Resistance in some Gram-negative species is intrinsic but there is also some enzyme destruction of the antibiotic by the production of a beta-lactamase (cephalosporinase) by some Gram-negative bacilli, although the cephalosporins tend to be less susceptible to the beta-lactamase produced by staphylococci.

Cefoxitin

This is a semi-synthetic member of a group of beta-lactam antibiotics, the *cephamycins*, that resemble the cephalosporins. As it is almost totally resistant to all beta-lactamases cefoxitin has a broad-spectrum effect. It is effective against *Escherichia coli*, *Proteus* spp and *Bacteroides* spp, as well as against pathogens normally sensitive to the cephalosporins.

The aminoglycosides

These include *streptomycin*, *neomycin*, *framycetin*, *kanamycin*, *amikacin*, *gentamicin* and *tobramycin*. They are active against many Gram-negative bacilli and staphylococci but not against streptococci or against anaerobic bacteria.

Streptomycin

Antibacterial spectrum and uses. This drug has a high degree of activity against Gram-negative bacilli, but the newer aminoglycosides such as kanamycin and gentamicin are now used more frequently for such infections. Streptomycin is still important in the treatment of tuberculosis and can be used also in synergistic combination with penicillin or ampicillin in the treatment of infective endocarditis caused by *Streptococcus faecalis* and the viridans streptococci, although combinations of other penicillins and aminoglycosides have been recommended.

Neomycin and framycetin

Antibacterial spectrum and uses. These antibiotics are similar in most respects. They are too toxic for systemic use and are therefore applied topically; both can be used to suppress nasal carriage of *Staphylococcus aureus* and they may be useful for superficial infections caused by coliform bacilli. Neomycin, because it is poorly absorbed from the gut, can be given before intestinal surgery in an attempt to suppress growth of organisms in the intestine. Whether attempted preoperative 'sterilisation' of the intestine is of any benefit is open to serious doubt.

Kanamycin

Antibacterial spectrum and uses. As with neomycin it can be used to suppress the aerobic Gram-negative bowel flora preoperatively. It is effective in treatment of severe systemic infections by Gram-negative bacilli, particularly those caused by *Proteus* spp, and is of considerable use in the treatment of those severe urinary tract infections that may be associated with septicaemia.

Amikacin

This is a derivative of kanamycin but with a slightly broader spectrum of action, in that *Pseudomonas* spp are sensitive to it.

Gentamicin

Antibacterial spectrum and uses. This drug has a broader spectrum of activity than the other aminoglycosides and a lower inhibitory concentration is required against *Escherichia, Klebsiella, Proteus* and *Salmonella* spp; it is more effective against *Pseudomonas* spp and *Staphylococcus aureus*. In serious pseudomonas infections it may be given in combination with carbenicillin. It is also given in combination with penicillin or ampicillin in the treatment of infective endocarditis caused by viridans streptococci or *Streptococcus faecalis*.

Tobramycin

Antibacterial spectrum and uses. This recently introduced antibiotic may prove more effective than gentamicin in the treatment of pseudomonas infection,

Mode of action. All aminoglycosides are bacteriocidal and act by inhibiting protein synthesis. They have some serious toxic effects on the eighth cranial nerve and kidney related to the blood levels.

Resistance. Mutation produces ribosomes that are no longer inhibited by the drug. R-factor resistance, by production of enzymes that inactivate aminoglycosides, occurs in enterobacteria. There can be cross resistance but this is not complete within the group.

The tetracyclines

These comprise a group of closely-related antibiotics that include *tetracycline*, *chlortetracycline*, *oxytetracycline*, *doxycycline*, *minocycline* and *demethylchlortetracycline*. Their antibacterial activity is very similar and there is little to choose amongst them.

Antibacterial spectrum and uses. Their spectrum of activity is broad. They are effective against Gram-positive and Gram-negative bacteria, both aerobes and anaerobes, as well as against mycoplasmas, chlamydiae and *Coxiella burneti*, although many *Bacteroides* spp are now resistant. They are commonly used in acute exacerbations of chronic bronchitis.

Mode of action. The tetracyclines are bacteriostatic and inhibit protein synthesis by prokaryotic ribosomes.

Resistance. Acquired resistance is common now in bacteria that were previously sensitive such as *Staphylococcus aureus*, *Streptococcus pyogenes* and pneumococci.

Chloramphenicol

Antibacterial spectrum and uses. A broad-spectrum antibiotic, chloramphenicol is effective against most pathogenic bacteria, with the exception of *Pseudomonas* spp, but because of its toxic side effects on the bone marrow and its possible role in causing circulatory collapse in infants its use must be severely limited to certain infections, notably *Haemophilus influenzae* meningitis in children and the acute stages of typhoid fever; for both of these infections it is the drug of choice.

Mode of action. Chloramphenicol produces its bacteriostatic effect by inhibiting protein synthesis.

Resistance. Resistance to chloramphenicol is present on the R-factors of many coliform bacilli particularly in countries where it is still widely available without prescription.

Erythromycin

Antibacterial spectrum and uses. Like benzyl penicillin this is a narrow-spectrum drug, active primarily against Gram-positive organisms such as beta-haemolytic streptococci, pneumococci and some *Staphylococcus aureus*, Gram-negative anaerobes and clostridia. It is not effective against the enterobacteria and most other Gram-negative bacilli although it is active against neisseriae, *Haemophilus influenzae, Bordetella pertussis* and many strains of *Bacteroides* spp; it has also an effect against some chlamydiae and rickettsiae. It is particularly useful however in the treatment of patients who are hypersensitive to penicillin.

Mode of action. This is mainly bacteriostatic, though high doses may be bacteriocidal. It acts on bacterial ribosomes to inhibit protein synthesis.

Resistance. In *Staphylococcus aureus*, streptococci and pneumococci this arises rather easily by mutation, though resistant strains usually disappear if the drug is discontinued for a period.

The lincomycins

Lincomycin and *clindamycin* are similar in many ways to *erythromycin* in antibacterial spectrum, mode of action and resistance. Cross resistance occurs amongst these drugs. *Clindamycin* is the newer, better absorbed and more active drug and has a greater effect against anaerobes. Both are useful in the treatment of infections caused by Gram-positive aerobes, such as *Staphylococcus aureus*, and because of very good penetration and diffusion to tissues such as bone they are recommended for the treatment of acute and chronic osteomyelitis. A combination of gentamicin and clindamycin may be invaluable in blind treatment of serious undiagnosed infection.

Fusidic acid

Antibacterial spectrum and uses. Fusidic acid is effective against many Gram-positive cocci, Gram-negative cocci and Gram-positive bacilli but its outstanding action is against *Staphylococcus aureus*. It has been used successfully in acute and chronic forms of staphylococcal disease.

Mode of action. Fusidic acid inhibits protein synthesis.

Resistance. Resistance to the drug is plasmid-borne.

The polypeptides

Antibacterial spectrum and uses. These antibiotics are nearly all too toxic for systemic use but can be of value as topical agents in infections of the eye, ear and burns. *Colistin* (polymyxin E), the only member that can be given systemically, is active against *Pseudomonas aeruginosa*. *Bacitracin*, a peptide antibiotic, is too toxic for systemic use but is sometimes included in mixtures of antibiotics for topical use. It is used in the laboratory, incorporated in a paper disk, as a screening test for *Streptococcus pyogenes*.

Metronidazole

Most anaerobic infections, with the possible exception of clostridial infections, can be treated effectively with this drug. Vincent's infection, trichomoniasis and amoebic dysentery can also be treated with this agent.

Rifampicin

In combination with other antituberculous drugs rifampicin can be used successfully in the treatment of tuberculosis. A combination with another drug is desirable because resistance develops rapidly unless this is prevented by the presence of another active drug.

FURTHER READING

Garrod, L. P., Lambert, H. P. & O'Grady, F. (1975) *Antibiotic and Chemotherapy*. Edinburgh: Churchill Livingstone.

Stokes, E. J. (1975) *Clinical Bacteriology*. London: Arnold.

Watt, P. J. (1969) *The Control of Chemotherapy*. Edinburgh: Churchill Livingstone.

6

Infections of the central nervous system and locomotor system

CENTRAL NERVOUS SYSTEM

Defences against infection

The cerebrospinal fluid (CSF) does not contain any effective antibacterial substances and since there are no other local defences infection rapidly becomes generalised when a pyogenic organism gains access to the subarachnoid space and the cerebrospinal fluid, by direct extension or via the blood.

Potential pathogens (see Fig. 6.1)

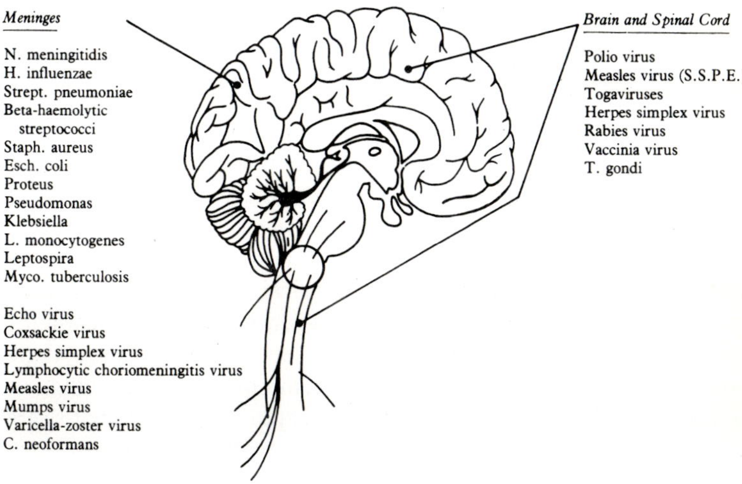

Fig. 6.1 Potential pathogens of the central nervous system

Acute pyogenic meningitis

Bacterial aetiology

Table 6.1 shows the causes of acute bacterial meningitis in England, Wales and Ireland in 1973 and 1976. The aetiology of acute pyogenic (acute bacterial) meningitis has a certain relationship with the age of the patient; coliform bacilli and group B streptococci (*Streptococcus agalactiae*) are common causes in the neonate, *Haemophilus influenzae* and *Neisseria meningitidis* in children up to five years of age, *Neisseria meningitidis* in older children, adolescents and adults, and *Streptococcus pneumoniae* in adults.

Table 6.1 Causes of bacterial meningitis (England, Wales and Ireland 1973 and 1976)

Organism	Number of cases for the year 1973	(with deaths) 1976
Neisseria meningitidis	756 (47)	571 (45)
Haemophilus influenzae	317 (9)	320 (17)
Streptococcus pneumoniae	221 (52)	239 (55)
Escherichia coli	78 (27)	76 (2)
Proteus spp	8 (3)	12 (3)
Pseudomonas spp	5 (1)	20 (4)
Streptococcus spp	43 (16)	51 (22)
Staphylococcus spp	36 (8)	64 (8)
Mycobacterium tuberculosis	20 (4)	23 (6)
Listeria monocytogenes	17 (3)	13 (4)
Others	21 (5)	12 (3)
All	1522 (175)	1401 (189)

Pathogenesis and epidemiology

Neonatal meningitis. Although in former years this was commonly caused by *Streptococcus pyogenes* and *Staphylococcus aureus*, coliform bacilli have been important causes in the last two decades. In recent years, group B streptococci have been responsible for many cases of neonatal meningitis and at present they rival the coliform organisms in being the most common causative agents. Coliform meningitis often results from congenital deformities such as spina bifida, and the sources of the organisms can be the genitourinary tract, lungs or umbilicus. Two forms of group B streptococcal meningitis are recognised; the *early-onset* form that occurs within 36 hours of birth and in which infection is contracted from the cervicovaginal canal of the mother, and the *late-onset* form that does not usually occur until 10 days or more after birth and which may be nosocomial in origin.

Haemophilus meningitis. Although adult cases have been described this occurs almost exclusively in young children between the ages of three months and five years. Protection before three months is provided by maternal antibody and after five years by acquired immunity. Infection is spread by the bloodstream from some focus such as an upper respiratory tract infection. Capsulate organisms of Pittman's type b are most commonly responsible for these infections.

Meningococcal meningitis. Meningococci enter the body via the nasopharynx where they may either produce a localised inflammatory reaction or remain quiescent. There are two main theories as to how they reach the meninges: (1) that they spread by direct extension along the spaces between the sheath and the branches of the olfactory nerve that pierce the cribriform plate; and (2) the more likely theory, that the organisms invade the bloodstream and either produce a transient bacteriaemia or multiply in the blood and cause metastatic lesions elsewhere in the body, in the skin, adrenal glands, joints and meninges. Nine groups of meningococci (A–D; X, Y, Z, Z^1, W135) are recognised; group B is the most common in the United Kingdom.

Infection is most readily spread in conditions of close household contact, although a striking feature of any epidemic is the low morbidity; fewer than 1 per cent of people at risk are infected. An epidemic may be heralded by a rise in the normal 5–10 per cent carrier rate in the community but an increase in the carrier rate does not necessarily mean that meningococcal infection will occur.

Pneumococcal meningitis. This may be caused either by septicaemic spread secondary to conditions such as lobar pneumonia or otitis media, or by direct infection from the paranasal sinuses following injury to the skull. Infection after injury is a particularly serious form of meningitis in the adult and carries a high mortality rate in elderly patients.

Meningitis due to other bacteria. These include *Staphylococcus aureus* and *Streptococcus pyogenes.* They reach the meninges either via the bloodstream, by direct extension from the ear or paranasal sinuses, or directly from the exterior after trauma.

Tuberculous meningitis. This occurs in a particularly severe form in young children and is probably secondary to a tuberculous focus elsewhere in the body, although this often cannot be located. The bacilli reach the meninges via the bloodstream.

Laboratory diagnosis of meningitis

Laboratory diagnosis is made by the isolation and identification of the specific organism from the blood and cerebrospinal fluid and in some cases by the detection of antigen in the CSF by techniques such as counterimmunoelectrophoresis. Changes occur in the cerebrospinal fluid depending on whether the aetiology is acute pyogenic, tuberculous or viral (see Table 6.2).

Blood cultures are particularly useful in the diagnosis of meningitis and may be positive in approximately 50 per cent of cases. About 5 ml

Table 6.2 The cerebrospinal fluid in meningitis

	Normal	Acute pyogenic	Tuberculous	Aseptic
Appearance	Clear	Turbid	Clear or opalescent	Usually clear
Total protein	0.15–0.4 g/l	Greatly increased; (10-fold and more)	Increased	Normal
Sugar	2.6–4.3 mmol/l	Greatly reduced or absent	Reduced	Normal
Cell count	0–3 lymphocytes per cu mm	Greatly increased; [a]NPNLS	Increased; mainly lymphocytes but some NPNLS	Increased; lymphocytes

[a]Neutrophil polymorphonuclear leucocytes

of cerebrospinal fluid is removed by lumbar puncture and a cell count made. The fluid is centrifuged and Gram films are made from the deposit (Ziehl-Neelsen if tuberculous meningitis is suspected). Microscopy may be sufficient to indicate the diagnosis and to allow chemotherapy to commence but cultures are also made on blood agar, 'chocolate' (heated blood) agar and on New York City medium which is selective for neisseriae. They are incubated up to 24 hours in an atmosphere of 10 per cent carbon dioxide. Biochemical and/or serological tests confirm the identity of the organism. For tuberculous meningitis Löwenstein-Jensen slopes are set up and guinea pigs may be inoculated.

Prophylaxis

This applies particularly to meningococcal meningitis. Chemoprophylaxis has been attempted for many years but without a great deal of success. Formerly sulphonamides were used to remove the organisms from the nasopharynx and were effective until a large proportion of meningococci became resistant. The penicillins which are effective and indeed essential in treating the clinical case are ineffective in eliminating the carrier state. Other antimicrobial drugs such as tetracyclines including minocycline and rifampicin have been used with varying degrees of success.

Resistance to meningococcal meningitis is related to the possession of antibody, and the possibility of producing immunity is currently under study in America where purified carbohydrate vaccine prepared from group C strains has been found to be protective.

Treatment

Chemotherapy will depend on the nature of the organism and laboratory sensitivity tests, but in general benzyl penicillin is a useful agent; chloramphenicol is used for the treatment of *Haemophilus* meningitis. Sulphonamides are now less widely used empirically because of the problem of increasing bacterial resistance, particularly in meningococci.

Cerebral abscess

Bacterial aetiology

The following bacteria can cause this condition: *Streptococcus milleri*, *beta-haemolytic streptococci*, *Streptococcus pneumoniae*, *Staphylococcus aureus*, *Haemophilus influenzae*, coliform bacilli, *Bacteroides* spp, *Fusobacterium* spp, *Veillonella* and other anaerobic cocci. Infections are often mixed.

Pathogenesis and epidemiology

Abscess formation can occur via the bloodstream or as the result of direct extension into the brain. The sources of infection vary and include otitis media, sinusitis and metastatic spread from chest infection. Infection may also follow dental, abdominal or neurological surgery and may occur after head injuries. Temporal lobe or cerebellar hemisphere abscesses are associated with otitis media and mastoiditis and frontal lobe abscesses with infection of the ethmoidal, sphenoidal and frontal sinuses. Frontal lobe abscesses are also a complication of acute and chronic dental infection. The mortality rate from brain abscess is about 40 per cent despite treatment.

Laboratory diagnosis

It is most important to obtain pus and make a Gram film in addition to culturing the specimen both aerobically and anaerobically.

Treatment

Where practicable excision of abscesses is mandatory and antibiotics must be given. The penicillin group and gentamicin are widely used, and metronidazole should always be considered because of the frequent associations of *Bacteroides fragilis* and other anaerobic bacteria with cerebral abscess.

Botulism

Bacterial aetiology

Botulism is a severe and frequently fatal form of food poisoning caused by the consumption of food containing preformed toxin of *Clostridium botulinum*. Six main types of organisms (A–F) are recognised on the basis of their antigenically distinct toxins.

Pathogenesis and epidemiology

Clostridium botulinum, an anaerobic spore-forming Gram-positive bacillus, is a widely distributed saprophyte in soil, fruits, vegetables leaves, animal manure and sea mud. Human cases of botulism are rare and have been traced to a variety of foods such as fish, ham, sausage, home-canned meats and home-bottled vegetables such as peas and beans. Man is mainly affected by type A but a few cases of type E have been traced to preserved fish. The toxin affects the cholinergic system and seems to block release of acetylcholine. Neurotoxic effects include oculomotor and pharyngeal paralysis, dysphagia and respiratory failure.

Laboratory diagnosis

Suspected food should be examined bacteriologically and Gram-stained films can be examined for sporing Gram-positive bacilli; *Clostridium botulinum* can be isolated using anaerobic techniques; food can be tested for toxin and the patient's blood screened by animal inoculation and toxin neutralisation tests.

Prophylaxis

Home preservation of foodstuffs such as meat, fish, and vegetables such as peas and beans should be avoided, although acidic fruits can be bottled safely since *Clostridium botulinum* does not grow at a low pH. A prophylactic dose of polyvalent antitoxin may be given to asymptomatic persons who are thought to have ingested the toxin.

Treatment

Polyvalent antitoxin is of little value once symptoms have appeared and general supportive treatment is all that can be offered to such patients.

Tetanus

Bacterial aetiology

Clostridium tetani.

Pathogenesis and epidemiology

Tetanus is the result of contamination of a wound with *Clostridium tetani* spores, frequently from manured soil, contaminated dust or clothing. Germination of the spores in a wound depends on reduced oxygen tension which can occur in any devitalised tissue and which may also be produced if aerobes multiply concomitantly in the wound. Infection remains localised although the clinical condition is caused by the effects of a potent diffusible toxin on the nervous system. The toxin travels by way of the motor nerves to the brain and spinal cord and interferes with the transmission of motor nerve impulses.

Although tetanus is commonly associated with deep wounds it can nevertheless result from superficial abrasions, including scratches and rose-thorn pricks.

Laboratory diagnosis

Gram films can be made from the wound exudate and examined for *drum-stick bacilli.* Special stains can reveal the characteristic terminal spore. The bacilli grow well on blood-containing media under strict anaerobic conditions. Biochemical tests can confirm their identity and animal inoculation can test for toxigenicity of the organism.

Prophylaxis

1. *Prevention of germination of tetanus spores.* This includes prompt and thorough wound toilet and surgical debridement if required.
2. *Provision of sufficient antitoxin to neutralise any tetanus toxin that may be produced.* This can be done either by giving (a) a booster dose of tetanus toxoid to those already actively immunised or (b) anti-tetanus serum (ATS) to those not actively immunised. *Human anti-tetanus globulin (ATG)* should be used in preference to ATS because of the risk of hypersensitivity reactions in patients given horse antiserum. ATG is freely available in the United Kingdom but this situation may not apply in developing countries. Combined active-passive immunisation must be given to the non-immune person; this gives immediate passive protection by the ATG while active immunity is developing.
3. *Prevention of multiplication (and therefore toxin production) of the vegetative bacilli.* This can be achieved by giving prophylactic antibiotics (and can replace 2b), although the use of both procedures is recommended.

Treatment
As well as general measures such as the use of muscle relaxants, sedation and artifical ventilation, antitoxin can be given although this is of little use if the toxin has become fixed to the tissues. Those who recover from tetanus require a course of active immunisation because the disease does not produce immunity.

THE LOCOMOTOR SYSTEM

Defences against infection
In the joint these include the synovial membrane and its cells which are specialised macrophages with a highly phagocytic action. Synovial fluid contains a few mononuclear cells, some complement and lysozyme.

Potential pathogens (see Fig. 6.2)

Acute septic arthritis

Bacterial aetiology
Bacteria commonly associated with this infection are *Staphylococcus*

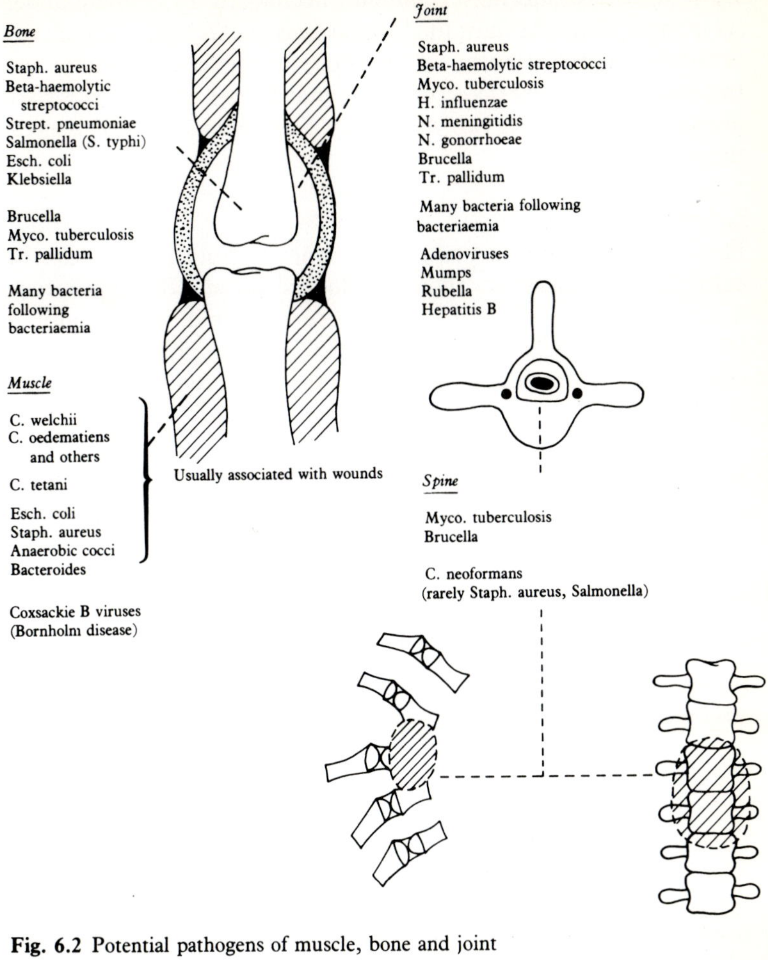

Fig. 6.2 Potential pathogens of muscle, bone and joint

aureus, Haemophilus influenzae, beta-haemolytic streptococci and neisseriae, together with rarer causes such as *Brucella* spp and *Salmonella* spp.

Pathogenesis and epidemiology

Infection can occur by: (1) penetrating injury through the joint capsule; (2) secondary direct spread from a nearby focus of infection such as osteomyelitis; and (3) haematogenous spread to the capillary network in the synovial membrane and thence to the joint. The knee joints are most frequently affected, then the hip and ankle.

Sources of septic arthritis are numerous and include sepsis of the skin, nasopharynx, sinuses, lung, peritoneum and genital tract. Acute septic arthritis occurs most commonly in children. In an infant under six months of age the most likely organisms are *Staphylococcus aureus* or Gram-negative organisms of faecal origin; between six months and two years of age *Staphylococcus aureus* and *Haemophilus influenzae* are predominant, and over two years of age *Staphylococcus aureus* is again the major cause.

Laboratory diagnosis

Blood cultures must be taken and synovial fluid should also be cultured. A primary site should be looked for and the appropriate material cultured. Synovial fluid appears turbid and creamy if infected, and will have a great increase in neutrophil polymorphs. (Exudate in rheumatoid arthritis looks turbid but no bacteria can be cultured).

Treatment

This will be dictated by the organism isolated and the results of sensitivity testing.

Acute osteomyelitis

Bacterial aetiology

Predominant bacteria are *Staphylococcus aureus,* beta-haemolytic streptococci, *Streptococcus pneumoniae* and Gram-negative bacilli, including *Haemophilus influenzae*, *Escherichia coli* and *Salmonella* spp. Tuberculosis and syphilis of bone can also occur.

Pathogenesis and epidemiology

This infection can occur in any bone and results from haematogenous spread from a septic focus (perhaps quite minor) elsewhere in the body. The femur is most frequently affected, followed by the tibia, then the foot bones, humerus, fibula and pelvis. It is most common under the age of 12 and affects males more often than females.

Laboratory diagnosis

Blood cultures must be taken and if pus can be obtained this should also be processed. As with septic arthritis the primary site should be sought and material cultured. Treatment has to be started as soon as possible, probably before the results of culture are known and a 'best guess' approach may have to be adopted. As over 90 per cent of cases are caused by *Staphylococcus aureus,* cloxacillin or another anti-staphylococcal agent is the treatment of choice.

FURTHER READING

Adams, E. B., Laurence, D. R. & Smith, J. W. G. (1969) *Tetanus*. Oxford: Blackwell Scientific Publications.

Christie, A. B. (1974) *Infectious Diseases: Epidemiology and Clinical Practice*. Edinburgh: Churchill Livingstone.

Cruickshank, R., Duguid, J. P., Marmion, B. P. & Swain, R. H. A. (1973) *Medical Microbiology*. Edinburgh: Churchill Livingstone.

Davies, P. A. (1977) Neonatal bacterial meningitis. *British Journal of Hospital Medicine*, **18**, 425–434.

Garrod, L. P., Lambert, H. P. & O'Grady, F. (1975) *Antibiotic and Chemotherapy*. Edinburgh: Churchill Livingstone.

7

Infections of the mouth

Normal flora

The many varied species of organisms that comprise the normal flora of the mouth are listed in Table 7.1. Numbers and species of organisms vary from region to region.

Table 7.1 The normal flora of the mouth

(i) *Organisms generally present that constitute a major fraction of the oral flora*
Viridans streptococci (*Streptococcus salivarius, sanguis, mutans, milleri, mitis*).
Corynebacterium spp
Neisseria spp
Haemophilus spp
Veillonella spp
Lactobacillus spp
Leptotrichia spp
Actinomyces spp
Bacteroides spp
Bacterionema spp
Eikenella spp

(ii) *Organisms generally present that constitute a minor fraction of the oral flora*
Anaerobic cocci
Streptococcus pneumoniae
Staphylococcus spp
Fusobacterium spp
Spirochaetes (*Borrelia* and *Treponema*)
Campylobacter spp
Clostridium spp
Mycoplasma spp
Candida spp
Nocardia spp

(iii) *Organisms that are transient or associated with the carrier state in the mouth*
Beta-haemolytic streptococci
Staphylococcus spp
Neisseria meningitidis
Coliform organisms
Corynebacterium diphtheriae
Protozoa
Viruses

Table 7.2 Mean percentages of cultivable organisms in the adult oral cavity (Socransky and Manganiello, 1971)

	Gingival crevice area	Dental plaque	Tongue	Saliva
Gram-positive facultative cocci	28.8	28.2	44.8	46.2
Streptococci	27.1	27.9	38.3	41.0
Strept. salivarius	ND	ND	8.2	4.6
Enterococci	7.2	ND	ND	1.3
Staphylococci	1.7	0.3	6.5	4.0
Gram-positive anaerobic cocci	7.4	12.6	4.2	13.0
Gram-negative facultative cocci	0.4	0.4	3.4	1.2
Gram-negative anaerobic cocci	10.7	6.4	16.0	15.9
Gram-positive facultative rods	15.3	23.8	13.0	11.8
Gram-positive anaerobic rods	20.2	18.4	8.2	4.8
Gram-negative facultative rods	1.2	ND	3.2	2.3
Gram-negative anaerobic rods	16.1	10.4	8.2	4.8
Fusobacterium spp	1.9	4.1	0.7	0.3
B. melaninogenicus	4.7	ND	0.2	ND
V. sputorum	3.8	1.3	2.2	2.1
Other *Bacteroides* spp	5.6	4.8	5.1	2.4
Spirochaetes	1.0	ND	ND	ND

ND = not detected

Table 7.2 shows the percentages of cultivable organisms from the gingival crevice area, dental plaque, tongue and saliva, and Table 7.3 compares the proportions of bacteria that can be isolated from saliva and from 14-day-old plaque.

Table 7.3 Proportions of bacterial groups in dental plaque (14 days) and saliva

	Dental plaque (14 days) %	Saliva %
Gram-positive cocci	41	61
Gram-negative cocci	7	16
Gram-positive rods	41	18
Gram-negative rods	10	3
Spirillum spp	1	2
Spirochaetes	±	0

Defences against infection

The oral cavity represents a very sophisticated ecosystem and there are many factors that contribute to the prevention of infection (see Table 7.4).

Table 7.4 Defences against infection in the mouth

Anatomical factors
Morphology of the teeth and their spatial relationship
Intact keratinised oral mucosa
Tongue movements
Salivary flow and swallowing reflex

Salivary factors
Lysozyme from salivary glands, crevicular exudate and polymorphonuclear leucocytes
Thiocyanate-dependent factors
Lactoferrin
pH
Glucolytic activity of epithelial cells
Microbial antagonism
Normal flora
Salivary glycoprotein
Leucocytes from the gingival crevice
Immunoglobulins (IgA and secretory IgA, IgG and IgM from the salivary glands; IgG, IgA and IgM from the crevicular exudate)

In addition to these specific factors there are also general factors such as dental hygiene, the presence or absence of fluoride in drinking water, the nutritional status and general health of the host.

Potential pathogens (see Fig. 7.1)

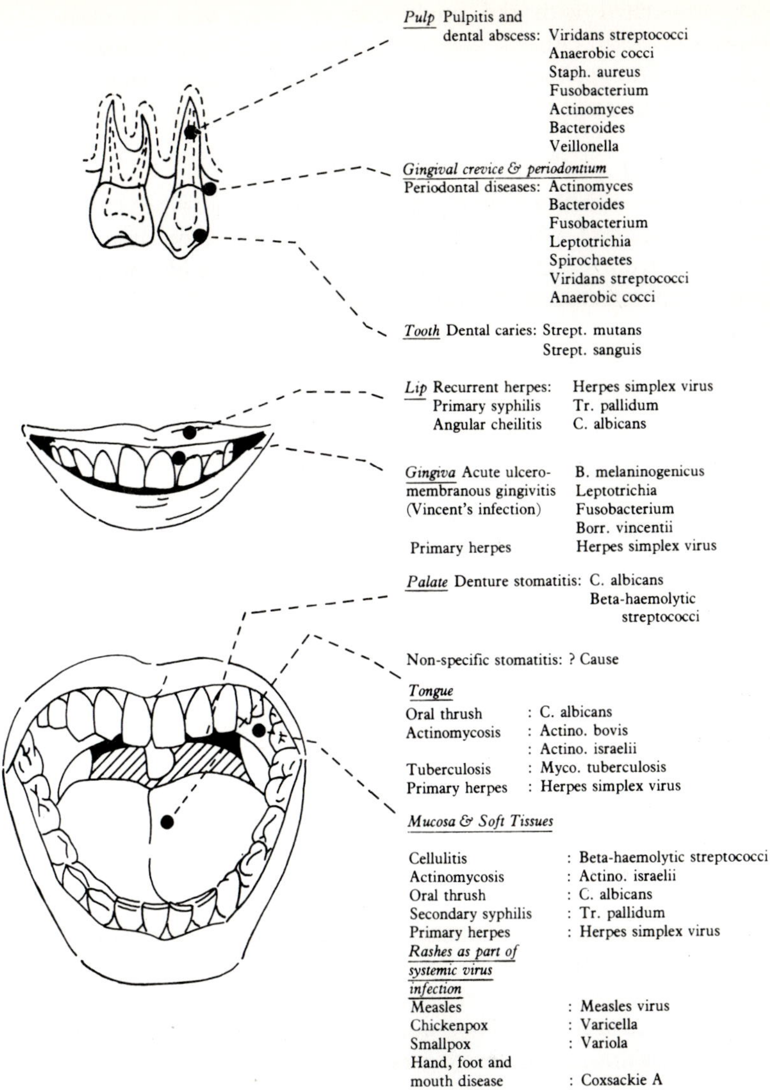

Fig. 7.1 Potential pathogens of the oral cavity

DENTAL CARIES

Bacterial aetiology

Bacteria, a susceptible host and a cariogenic diet are the three essentials for the production of caries. Viridans streptococci, chiefly *Streptococcus mutans* and to a lesser extent *Streptococcus sanguis*, are closely associated with the production of caries and are early colonisers of teeth. Other acidogenic bacteria including *Actinomyces* and *Lactobacillus* spp may contribute to the progression of caries, but are far less important than the viridans streptococci.

Pathogenesis and epidemiology
Rats and hamsters with a normal oral flora develop caries when fed on a diet rich in sucrose, whereas germ-free animals fed on the same diet remain free from caries. These animals however readily develop lesions when infected orally with a pure culture of *Streptococcus mutans*.

Dental plaque
This is a soft, often whitish, adherent deposit that forms on a tooth surface. Although plaque forms particularly after the abandonment of dental hygiene it is a constant factor in all mouths. It comprises a mucopolysaccharide matrix in which extracellular material, squamous cells and bacteria are embedded. Plaque is a dynamic entity and its bacterial composition, quite different from that of saliva changes constantly. (Tables 7.2, 7.3).

Plaque

Initial composition
Gram-positive cocci, *Neisseria, Nocardia* and some Gram-positive bacilli. Colonisation of a clean tooth surface in contact with saliva commences within an hour.

0–2 days. There is a very rapid rise in numbers of Gram-positive cocci to about 90 per cent of the total bacterial count.

2–4 days. An increase in filamentous forms, Gram-negative bacilli and Gram-negative cocci occurs. At this stage Gram-positive cocci constitute a lower percentage of the overall flora of plaque. Their numbers do not decrease but other organisms proliferate greatly.

7 days. There is a further increase in filamentous forms, Gram-negative bacilli, vibrios and *Actinomyces*.

14 days. Filamentous forms, Gram-negative bacilli, Gram-positive bacilli, vibrios and spirochaetes are predominant.

21 days. Many bacteria, particularly in the deeper layers of plaque, are now dead due to lack of nutritional substances and the presence of toxicity factors.

Supragingival plaque is associated with *dental caries, subgingival plaque* with *periodontal disease*.

Production of dental caries

There are two main theories of caries production: (1) acidogenic and (2) proteolytic. The *acidogenic theory*, the more probable, postulates that the initial lesion is a breach of the enamel caused by products of bacterial metabolism, notably of *Streptococcus mutans* and *Streptococcus sanguis*. These streptococci produce large amounts of extracellular polysaccharide, particularly dextran from sucrose, and this enables bacteria to adhere to the teeth. Other bacteria can thereafter contribute to the progression of caries. These include other viridans streptococci which can store intracellular polysaccharide when there are sufficient carbohydrate supplies. When these become scarce the intracellular stores can be utilised ensuring continued production of acids. The *proteolytic theory* states that proteolysis is the initial event, followed by decalcification.

A third theory put forward is the *proteolysis-chelation* theory which postulates primary proteolytic digestion of the organic matrix with subsequent decalcification by chelation of calcium with products of proteolytic digestion, such as aminoacids.

Prophylaxis

Prophylaxis of caries includes general measures such as proper dental care and hygiene, suitable diet and fluoridation of water supplies. In recent years immunisation of monkeys with serotype C of *Streptococcus mutans* has been relatively successful but how far this will prove to be a practical proposition in humans remains to be seen.

Treatment

Antibiotics have no place in the treatment of caries and once the lesion is established reparative dental treatment is required.

PERIODONTAL DISEASE

Bacterial aetiology

In recent years identification of organisms involved in periodontal disease has become more firmly based and the association of a group of organisms, rather than one or two particular species, is now recognised. These include *Actinomyces, Fusobacterium, Bacteroides, Leptotrichia*, spirochaetes, vibrios, viridans streptococci, anaerobic cocci and *Campylobacter*.

Pathogenesis and epidemiology

The periodontium comprises the gingivae, alveolar bone and periodontal membrane. Periodontal disease includes disease of any of the components and is a common human problem, particularly after adolescence. *Marginal gingivitis* is one of the commonest forms of periodontal disease and this may be acute or chronic.

The typical inflammatory response of periodontal tissues does not occur in the absence of bacteria and clinical and epidemiological observations, as well as animal studies, have provided firm evidence of the aetiological role of *subgingival plaque* in this disease.

Periodontal disease is produced by a combination of two main processes: (1) the effect on the tissues of bacterial products such as collagenase, hyaluronidase and neuraminidase, inducing an inflammatory reaction; and (2) the consequent production of immune responses, both humoral and cell-mediated, in the host.

Prophylaxis

Oral hygiene is of paramount importance in the prevention of this disease.

Treatment

Only in the most acute cases does antibiotic therapy have a place in the treatment of periodontal disease.

Pulp and periapical infections

Bacterial aetiology

Almost invariably infections of pulp and acute periapical abscesses are endogenous and many commensal bacteria may be involved; these are most commonly viridans streptococci and anaerobic cocci, staphylococci, *Neisseria, Haemophilus, Actinomyces, Fusobacterium, Bacteroides* and *Veillonella,* although it is often difficult to prove which particular species, or combinations of organisms, have actually produced the infection.

Pathogenesis and epidemiology

Infection of the pulp and periapical areas can occur by three pathways: (1) through the tubules of dentine, associated with caries; (2) by invasion along the periodontal membrane, associated with periodontal disease; and (3) through the bloodstream. Acute or chronic pulpitis can occur; in the acute form the inflammatory exudate in the pulp chamber can produce a rise in pressure causing spread of infection to the periapical tissues, either as cellulitis or as acute periapical abscess; a chronic lesion may result.

Laboratory diagnosis

Pus samples can be taken if practicable, and samples can also be taken from the root canal during operative procedures, using sterile paper points.

Treatment

Antibiotic therapy may be used to good effect in acute cases if drainage of the periapical area cannot be achieved. Once drainage has been established proper preparation of the root canal and adequate root filling measures are of paramount importance.

Oral candidiasis

Infections with *Candida* spp, including *Candida albicans, Candida stellatoidea* and *Candida tropicalis,* occur in both neonates and the elderly. In neonates the infection ('thrush') is acute and is contracted from the mother's genital tract. It is characterised by flaky, loosely-adherent membranes that cover the tongue, cheek and gums. Cross infection is common in neonatal nurseries.

In the elderly patient there is frequently some predisposing cause such as trauma, malignancy, endocrine disorders or antibiotic therapy. In these cases *Candida* spp, normally present as commensals in the mouth, assume the role of *opportunist pathogens.* There may be areas of white plaque or of erythematous inflammation with little plaque present. *Candida* spp produce *denture stomatitis* when trauma is caused by ill-fitting dentures and this is often associated with *angular cheilitis.*

AUMG

(Acute ulceromembranous gingivitis: Vincent's infection)

Bacterial aetiology

Two bacteria are commonly seen in films made from the necrotised gingival tissue; a spirochaete, *Borrelia vincenti* and a fusiform bacillus, *Leptotrichia buccalis* (formerly called *Fusobacterium fusiforme*). There is, however, increasing evidence that other members of the oral anaerobic flora, namely *Bacteroides melaninogenicus*, may play a part in the aetiology of the condition.

Pathology and epidemiology

This is an endogenous infection that causes an ulcerative gingivitis. Infection may be superimposed on trauma to the oral mucosa, on vitamin deficiencies and on other compromising factors such as blood dyscrasias. The disease is not transmissible.

Laboratory diagnosis

This depends on the following findings in stained films; pus cells,

Gram-negative spirochaetes (*Borrelia vincenti*) and Gram-negative fusiform bacilli. Cultural methods are not satisfactory.

Treatment

Metronidazole is the drug of choice. Penicillin is also effective.

FURTHER READING

Burnett, G. W. & Scherp, H. W. (1962) *Oral Microbiology and Infectious Disease.* Baltimore: Williams and Wilkins.

Melville, T. H. & Russell, C. (1975) *Microbiology for Dental Students.* London: Heinemann.

MacPhee, I. T. (1972) *Host Resistance to Commensal Bacteria.* Edinburgh: Churchill Livingstone.

8

Infections of the respiratory tract

Normal flora

Although the lower respiratory tract in health is sterile, several species of organisms colonise the upper respiratory tract, particularly the nose and throat. These are predominantly aerobes and include species of staphylococci, streptococci including pneumococci, corynebacteria, *Haemophilus* and neisseriae.

Defences against infection (see Table 8.1)

Table 8.1 Defences against infection in the respiratory tract

The vibrissae of the nose; these filter particles larger than 10–15 μm
Broncho-constriction
The cough reflex
Mucus glands and goblet cells
Ciliary action
Non-specific mucosal factors such as alpha antitrypsin, lactoferrin and lysozyme
Lymphatics of the bronchi and bronchioles
The alveolar macrophage system
Local humoral mucosal antibody (secretory IgA)
Bronchus-associated lymphoid aggregates
Local cell-mediated mucosal antibody

Potential pathogens (see Fig. 8.1)

Infection of the paranasal sinuses

This can be acute or chronic and is caused by pneumococci, *Haemophilus influenzae, Staphylococcus aureus,* beta-haemolytic streptococci and anaerobic cocci, bacteria that colonise adjacent areas. Bacterial infection occurs in association with obstruction resulting from mucosal oedema. Inflammation of the maxillary sinuses is common in uncomplicated virus infections of the upper respiratory tract.

Otitis media

Frequently otitis media is the result of direct spread of pathogens, namely pneumococci, *Haemophilus influenzae* and beta-haemolytic

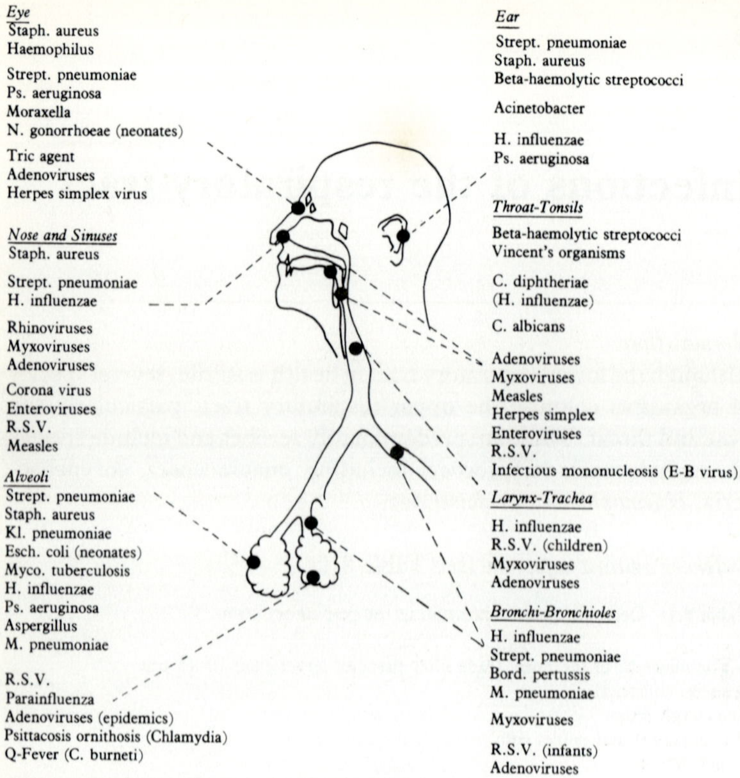

Fig. 8.1 Potential pathogens of the respiratory tract

streptococci, from the throat via the Eustachian tube. This infection can be acute or chronic and may be caused by viruses and mycoplasmas as well as bacteria. In the young the bacteria most frequently involved are pneumococci, *Haemophilus influenzae* and beta-haemolytic streptococci, whereas in older patients *Staphylococcus aureus*, pneumococci, and in chronic cases, coliform organisms, may be responsible.

Sore throat

Infective causes of sore throat

1. Prodromal stages of infectious diseases.
2. Diphtheria.
3. Acute ulceromembranous gingivitis (see Ch. 7).
4. 'Sore throat syndrome'.

Prodromal stages of infectious diseases

Several infectious diseases may cause sore throat before the appearance of rashes or other signs, including chicken pox, measles and meningitis.

Diphtheria

Bacterial aetiology. *Corynebacterium diphtheriae; gravis, intermedius* and *mitis* are the three main biotypes.

Pathogenesis and epidemiology. Diphtheria begins as an acute inflammatory condition of the upper respiratory tract, usually the throat, but sometimes the nasal cavity. The bacilli multiply there and produce a powerful exotoxin which diffuses through the body affecting the myocardium, adrenal glands and nerve endings. At the site of infection the inflammatory exudate and necrotic mucosal cells form a membrane that remains adherent to the throat and this may produce respiratory obstruction. Figure 8.2 shows the pattern of the disease during the last century. The carriage rate in the United Kingdom of toxigenic corynebacteria is now negligible due to the national immunisation programme.

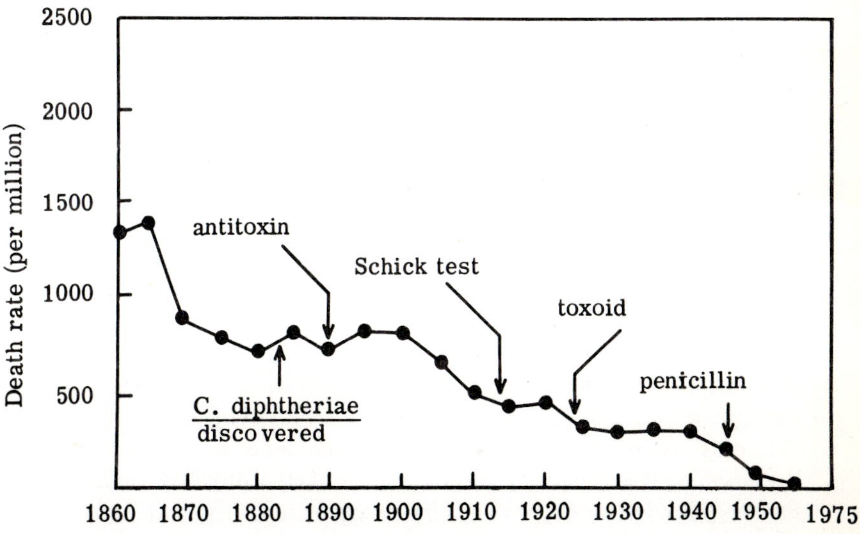

Fig. 8.2 Decline in incidence of diphtheria in the UK, 1860–1975

Laboratory diagnosis. A film of a throat swab should be made to exclude infections with Vincent's organisms and the swab should be inoculated on to a Loeffler slope to allow more rapid growth of the corynebacteria, and on to a selective medium of blood and potassium tellurite. An Albert-stained smear of the growth can be made from the Loeffler slope and examined after about ten hours for the presence of metachromatic granules. Agar-gel precipitation tests (Elek) and guinea-pig inoculation tests for toxigenicity will confirm the diagnosis.

Prophylaxis. Active immunisation is the most important measure. It is best to give diphtheria and tetanus toxoids with pertussis vaccine (*triple vaccine*) in three separate doses, beginning in the third month of life; there should be an interval of six to eight weeks and four to six months between the first and second and second and third injections respectively. A booster dose is given at school entry, omitting the pertussis element. An alum-adsorbed toxoid is the most effective measure when the antigen is used alone; toxoid-antitoxin floccules (TAF) can also be used. In older persons an intradermal *Schick* test should be done before giving immunisation and only those who are positive reactors to the toxin (local erythema and oedema which indicates little or no neutralising antitoxin) should be immunised.

Treatment. Large doses of antitoxin should be given as soon as possible although care is necessary as the antitoxin is produced in horses. Penicillin or erythromycin will eradicate most strains of *Corynebacterium diphtheriae* but antibiotics have no effect on toxin already produced. Patients and carriers should be isolated until nose and throat swabs are clear.

The sore throat syndrome (STS)

Bacterial aetiology. The STS is essentially an acute pharyngitis and/or an acute tonsillitis and is caused by bacteria, viruses and mycoplasmas. The bacteria are almost exclusively the Lancefield group A beta-haemolytic streptococci, *Streptococcus pyogenes*. Groups B, C and G may also be involved, but other bacteria such as staphylococci and *Haemophilus* organisms are only very rarely implicated. For all practical purposes a *bacterial* sore throat means a *streptococcal* sore throat, except in the compromised host in whom a variety of bacteria may produce infection. It is important to remember that only 30–40 per cent of cases of the STS are caused by streptococci; the remaining cases are most likely caused by viruses, such as adenovirus, rhinovirus, influenza, enterovirus and herpes viruses, or by *Mycoplasma pneumoniae*.

Pathogenesis and epidemiology. Sore throat is very common especially in the winter months but it is uncommon in the under-two-year olds and in the elderly. Its peak incidence is in the young school child who succumbs to the cross-infection hazards of the classroom, because of a poorly developed level and range of antibodies. It is much less common in the older school child, adolescent and young adult. Rarely a streptococcal sore throat can be contracted from eating contaminated food or drinking contaminated milk.

Laboratory diagnosis. Swabs should be sent off quickly to the laboratory because the longer the swab is in transit the greater are the chances of the organisms dying off (see Ch. 4). If delay in collection or in transit is anticipated swabs should be stored in the refrigerator, as this helps preserve the streptococci that cause sore throat. A sample of saliva may also be sent off in addition to the throat swab as many patients with streptococcal sore throat shed streptococci into the saliva.

Gram films of throat swabs are not helpful; swabs should be plated on blood media and on crystal violet. Many beta-haemolytic streptococci are more easily recognised after anaerobic incubation of culture plates. A bacitracin disk can help to differentiate group A from other beta-haemolytic streptococci (group A is mostly sensitive) but streptococcal grouping tests should be performed in doubtful cases.

The sore throat syndrome cannot be diagnosed on clinical evidence because symptoms and signs produced by both streptococci and viruses are similar, such as sore throat, pain on swallowing, tender, enlarged tonsillar lymph nodes, and pyrexia. The appearance of the throat is of little diagnostic help as non-infected throats can appear red, whereas *Streptococcus pyogenes* may be cultured from pale, normal-looking throats. An exudate over the tonsils is not necessarily an indication of streptococcal infection since many virus infections of the throat produce a similar exudate. The throat must be swabbed if an accurate diagnosis of the STS is to be made.

Treatment. Beta-haemolytic streptococci are universally sensitive to penicillin. Erythromycin is also a very useful drug in cases of penicillin hypersensitivity.

Acute epiglottitis: Acute laryngo-tracheo-bronchitis

Bacterial aetiology. Although viruses may be associated with both conditions, *Haemophilus influenzae, type b,* is the important causative organism.

Pathogenesis and epidemiology. Both conditions affect infants and young children and are frequently fulminating. Acute epiglottitis in young children due to *Haemophilus influenzae* may cause acute respiratory obstruction.

Laboratory diagnosis. In both infections there is a septicaemic phase and blood culture is frequently positive. Pharyngeal swabs may also be helpful.

Treatment. Because of the severity of both infections antibiotic therapy has to be on a 'best guess' basis, and penicillin or ampicillin may be used until the laboratory confirms the diagnosis.

Bronchitis

Bacterial aetiology. Two organisms predominate in acute exacerbations of chronic bronchitis, *Haemophilus influenzae* and *Streptococcus pneumoniae*.

Pathogenesis and epidemiology. Chronic bronchitis is a relapsing condition, common in the United Kingdom. Various factors are involved in addition to infection, namely smoking, previous lung damage, atmospheric pollution and cold damp weather.

Laboratory diagnosis. Sputum samples are examined although the diagnosis is easily made clinically. One of the main reasons for culture is to check on antibiograms of the probable pathogens, and to obtain reliable results it is essential that a proper sample of sputum is taken. Sputum may be homogenised prior to culture and examination of several samples of sputum is recommended.

Treatment. Each acute episode can be treated as it occurs or the patient can be put on a long-term course of antiobiotics over the winter months. In the latter event it is mandatory to check periodically the antibiotic sensitivities of any *Haemophilus* organisms isolated. Broad-spectrum antibiotics such as tetracyclines and ampicillin are useful in this condition but treatment must depend on sensitivity tests.

Whooping cough

Bacterial aetiology. Bordetella pertussis.

Pathogenesis and epidemiology. Infection is spread by direct droplet spray and in unprotected children the secondary attack rate in a family may be around 90 per cent. It is a serious disease in young children, especially females, and approximately 10 per cent of children under two years of age who contract the disease have to be admitted to hospital. The fatality rate in children under one year of age is 50 times higher than in one to four year olds and 100 times greater than in five to nine year olds. Immunity by infection or by immunisation is long lasting, and in so-called second attacks of whooping cough the possibility of an infection by *Bordetella parapertussis*, or by viruses should be considered. Figures 8.3 and 8.4 show whooping cough rates in Scotland and England and Wales over the last few years. Whooping cough occurs in epidemic proportions every few years.

Laboratory diagnosis. A pernasal swab or cough plate containing Bordet-Gengou or charcoal medium should be examined by the usual methods, and a swab may also be examined by immunofluorescence. With a good technique the organisms can be isolated from almost every case in the early stage of the disease if the patient is not on antibiotics. As time progresses isolation becomes more difficult but by the end of the second week serological tests such as agglutination

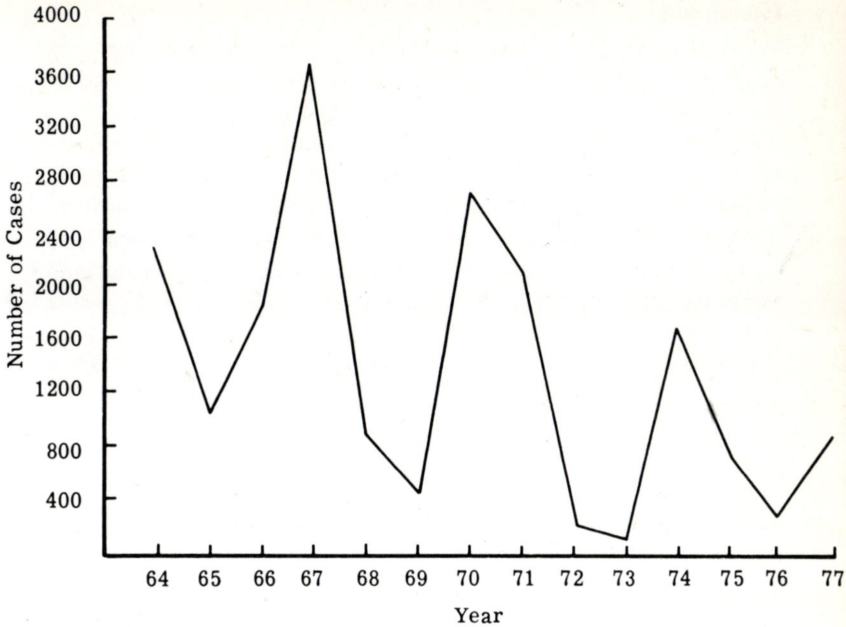

Fig. 8.3 Whooping cough in Scotland. Notification to the Registrar General, 1964–1977

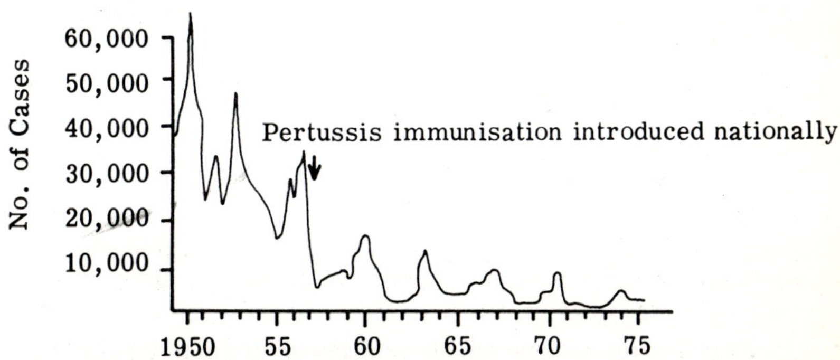

Fig. 8.4 Whooping cough. Quarterly notifications for England & Wales, 1950–75

and complement fixation tests can be performed.

Prophylaxis. Antibiotic prophylaxis has been suggested for children at risk from the infection who cannot be immunised.

Treatment. *Bordetella pertussis* is sensitive to many antibiotics *in vitro* but chemotherapy is generally unsatisfactory unless given very early in the infection, probably because the organisms are usually embedded in the deeper layers of the respiratory epithelium covered by a blanket of mucus and pus, where they can withstand any antibiotic siege.

Pneumonia

Bacterial aetiology. Lobar pneumonia is invariably caused by *Streptococcus pneumoniae* whereas *bronchopneumonia* can be caused by many pathogens.

Pathogenesis and epidemiology. By definition pneumonia is inflammation and consolidation of the lung substance and can be caused by physical and chemical agents as well as a host of microorganisms. The two main infective types are lobar and bronchopneumonia, although other types such as hypostatic and aspiration are described; these names refer rather to predisposing factors than to separate pathological entities.

Cross infection is the main means of production of lobar pneumonia, although infection may be caused by the pneumococci in the patient's own upper respiratory tract flora. There are over 80 pneumococcal serotypes but only a few are implicated in the majority of attacks. The pathogenesis involves invasion of the alveoli with subsequent deprivation of alveolar cells of adequate nutrition, resistance of the capsulate organisms to phagocytosis and the production of one or more exotoxins, such as pneumolysin.

In *bronchopneumonia* it is frequently difficult to determine the causative organism because of the multiplicity of bacteria but infection is usually endogenous and most frequently caused by *Streptococcus pneumoniae*, *Staphylococcus aureus* and *Haemophilus influenzae*. Coliform organisms are also commonly involved. The course of the disease is unpredictable and the response to treatment is frequently capricious, unlike lobar pneumonia. In the latter young adults are often affected whereas in bronchopneumonia it is the young and old who succumb.

In children bronchopneumonia may follow a viral infection of the upper respiratory tract such as measles, and in the old and debilitated staphylococcal bronchopneumonia can be a particularly serious sequel to influenza.

Patients with *cystic fibrosis* are very susceptible to respiratory tract infection because of viscid bronchial secretions which reduce the efficacy of the clearing mechanisms. *Staphylococcus aureus* and *Haemophilus influenzae* commonly cause infection as well as opportunist pathogens such as *Pseudomonas aeruginosa*.

Mycoplasma pneumoniae is occasionally responsible for a type of pneumonia that begins as a sore throat and general malaise and progresses to chest pain and a cough with scanty sputum.

Laboratory diagnosis. A properly taken sample of sputum must be sent to the laboratory. Blood culture may also be useful in diagnosis of lobar pneumonia. A complement fixation test is available for mycoplasma antibody.

Prophylaxis. This has been attempted by the use of vaccines containing prevalent pneumococcal types, and a high degree of protection can be obtained by these. It is not a practicable proposition on a large scale but is useful for people at special risk.

Treatment. Antibiotic treatment will depend on sensitivity tests but penicillins are commonly used with a high measure of success.

Legionnaires' disease

Bacterial aetiology. A Gram-negative, non-acid-fast bacillus.

Pathogenesis and epidemiology. An explosive outbreak of severe respiratory illness occurred in delegates attending an American Legion Convention in Philadelphia in 1976. Twenty nine of 182 cases were fatal. A retrospectively diagnosed outbreak also occurred in Benidorm in 1973.

The mode of spread of this infection is probably airborne although possibly from person to person; the source of the previously unrecognised bacterium is uncertain but it may be a commensal organism and searches are being made for it in bird and rodent populations and in dust. In the Philadelphia outbreak many of the staff in the hotels where the delegates stayed had raised antibody titres to the organisms, suggesting that exposure may have been intermittent over several years and that asymptomatic infection is common. There is also increasing recognition of non-pulmonary disease such as intestinal and hepatic disorders and encephalopathy.

Laboratory diagnosis. The organism produces a characteristic disease in guinea pigs and a characteristic death pattern in chick embryos after yolk-sac inoculation; it fails to grow on ordinary bacteriological media but does so on special Mueller-Hinton medium. Immunofluorescent techniques and serological tests are used in the diagnosis.

Treatment. No one antibiotic gave uniformly satisfactory results in treatment of the Philadelphia delegates although erythromycin and tetracyclines gave better results than others.

Respiratory tuberculosis

Bacterial aetiology. Mycobacterium tuberculosis is the causative agent; *Mycobacterium bovis* no longer causes disease in the United Kingdom.

Pathogenesis and epidemiology. The pathogenicity of tubercle bacilli depends on their ability to resist enzyme destruction when in the cytoplasm of macrophages. Intracellular growth occurs, the macrophages die and the bacilli either proceed to multiply extracellularly or, after ingestion by other macrophages, again intracellularly. Patients who recover naturally possess cell-mediated immunity and in addition usually have macrophages that have an enhanced ability to kill the organisms.

The most common form of primary (childhood) infection is the production of the primary complex, comprising (1) a focus (Ghon) of infection in the subpleural area, probably at the site of implantation of the infecting bacilli; and (2) involvement of the regional mediastinal glands draining the primary focus.

In the majority of cases infection clears up spontaneously causing no symptoms but in some cases a more generalised infection may be produced either by direct spread causing tuberculous bronchopneumonia, or by the haematogenous route causing miliary tuberculosis. The latter can affect many areas including the meninges, liver, kidneys, bones and joints.

Primary infection may occur via the intestinal tract if infected milk is drunk but this is now eradicated in the United Kingdom.

The post primary (secondary or adult) is the most common type of clinical tuberculosis. One or more lung lesions lead to caseation and cavitation and, if this involves the bronchial tree, open pulmonary tuberculosis results. Infection may be exogenous but may be caused by reactivation of a healed primary lesion. Such cases must be treated speedily and vigorously with appropriate antibiotics.

The mortality from tuberculosis has fallen dramatically since the middle of the last century. Notification rates are also considerably lowered, particularly in young children and young adults, formerly two of the most susceptible groups. At the present time tuberculosis is increasingly seen as an infection of the elderly.

Laboratory diagnosis. Tubercle bacilli are not commensal organisms and to isolate them from a patient is pathognomonic of the presence of tuberculous disease. Also because commensal or saprophytic mycobacteria are rarely found in the respiratory tract the finding of even one acid-fast bacillus on a sputum smear stained by the Ziehl-Neelsen method is substantial evidence of pulmonary tuberculosis. Such a provisional diagnosis is of immense importance as it allows chemotherapy to be started instantly without having to wait several weeks for the result of culture. A good sputum sample is best, failing which laryngeal swabs or gastric washings may be examined. Fluorescence microscopy may also be useful. Negative microscopical findings do not exclude the presence of tuberculosis as approximately 10^5 bacilli must be present in 1 ml sputum before positive microscopical findings can be reasonably expected.

Sputum should be cultured on egg-containing media in screw-cap containers to preserve moisture over the long incubation period of six veeks. Media in use are: (1) Löwenstein-Jensen (L-J); (2) modified

L-J media (IUT) which does not contain starch and is good for human type growth, although not for bovine; (3) sodium pyruvate medium, which is good for bovine strains, antibiotic-resistant human strains and atypical mycobacteria.

Guinea-pig inoculation may be useful.

Prophylaxis. This includes social measures, such as better nutrition. The use of selective radiography is helpful and segregation and chemotherapy of known cases is important. The use of the tuberculin test and administration of live attenuated vaccine (*BCG*) when required have also played a major role in the decrease in incidence of pulmonary tuberculosis.

The tuberculin test. The prevalence of tuberculosis can be measured by the use of the tuberculin test which when positive indicates that the person has at some time been infected by *Mycobacterium tuberculosis*, without necessarily having symptoms and signs of the disease. Tuberculin testing indicates a delayed hypersensitivity reaction which concomitantly indicates a degree of resistance to tuberculosis. *Old tuberculin* (*OT*), the specific tuberculo-protein, or a *purified protein derivative* (*PPD*), is introduced into the skin of the forearm by intradermal injection (Mantoux test), or by multiple puncture (Heaf and Tine tests).

Mantoux test. 0.1 ml of 1, 10 or 100 units of OT or PPD are injected intradermally. A positive test appears as an area of induration at least 5 mm in diameter, surrounded by an area of erythema.

Heaf test. The result is read at 3–7 days and the result is regarded as positive if four or more of the six puncture sites show indurated papules at least 1 mm in diameter. Grades 1–4 indicate degrees of reaction.

Tine test. A unit of four tines (prongs) is used. A positive result consists of induration of at least 2 mm in diameter in one or more puncture sites.

Whereas positive results indicate that the person has had previous contact with infection or has had BCG vaccine and has therefore a degree of protection to tuberculosis, it can also mean that the person is currently suffering from the disease. A negative result usually excludes the disease although false negative results can be obtained in acute forms of the disease such as tuberculous meningitis or in the early stages of tuberculosis.

Over the years the number of reactors has fallen markedly and it has been suggested that when the number falls to less than 1 per cent tuberculosis will have been controlled.

BCG (Bacille Calmette-Guérin) is named after the two Frenchmen who described this vaccine in 1921. It is a bovine strain of

Mycobacterium tuberculosis attenuated by repeated growth for many years on a bile-potato medium. The vaccine is given intradermally and should be offered to tuberculin-negative individuals who are at special risk and also to tuberculin-negative schoolchildren between 10–13 years of age. The tuberculin test should always first be performed because of the risk of severe local reactions if BCG is given to a tuberculin-positive person. Complications of vaccinations are rare.

Treatment. Various antibiotics are used, usually in combinations of three initially until sensitivities are known, and then in combinations of two. Isoniazid, para-amino salicylic acid (PAS), ethambutol, cycloserine, rifampicin, ethionamide and pyrazinamide are used. Because treatment has to be continued for many months it is mandatory that repeated sputum cultures are taken to ensure that they remain negative. There is a tendency for drug resistance to occur especially if they are used alone and this possibility must also be checked.

Lung abscess

Bacterial aetiology. Staphylococcus aureus, Streptococcus pyogenes, Streptococcus pneumoniae, various Gram-negative bacilli and anaerobic organisms such as *Bacteroides* spp, *Fusobacterium* spp and anaerobic cocci may be involved.

Pathogenesis and epidemiology. A lung abscess is usually secondary to some pre-existing condition such as pneumonia, the presence of foreign bodies, trauma and tumours. The most common group are those associated with bronchopneumonia, although they are rarer nowadays because of more effective therapy of the primary cause. Infected material is inhaled and obstructs the smaller bronchi and bronchioles producing atelectasis. Suppuration, necrosis and abscess formation occurs. Empyema or abscesses elsewhere in the body may follow.

Laboratory diagnosis. Sputum should be examined and pus should be processed if available but it is also most important to diagnose the primary cause.

Treatment. Surgical treatment and drainage may be required and antibiotic therapy depends on the results of antibiograms.

Empyema

This is a pleural abscess characterised by pus in the pleural space. An empyema is never primary and may be caused by: (1) extension of lobar pneumonia, bronchopneumonia, tuberculosis or lung abscess; (2) bacterial spread from the chest wall following thoracic surgery or trauma; (3) spread of infection from below the diaphragm, as in hepatic or subphrenic abscess. Pneumococci, staphylococci and *Haemophilus* organisms may be involved in spread from the lung, staphylococci and Gram-negative organisms from the chest wall, and coliform organisms and anaerobic cocci from under the diaphragm.

Pus must be aspirated and examined.

FURTHER READING

Christie, A. B. (1974) *Infectious diseases: Epidemiology and Clinical Practice*. Edinburgh: Churchill Livingstone.

Cruickshank, R., Duguid, J. P., Marmion, B. P. & Swain, R. H. A. (1973) *Medical Microbiology*. Edinburgh: Churchill Livingstone.

Dubos, R. J. & Hirsch, J. G. (1965) *Bacterial and Mycotic Infections of Man*. London: Pitman.

Garrod, L. P., Lambert, H. P. & O'Grady, F. (1975) *Antibiotic and Chemotherapy*. Edinburgh: Churchill Livingstone.

Horne, N. W. (1971) Epidemiology and control of tuberculosis. *British Journal of Hospital Medicine*, 5, 732–747.

Ross, P. W. (1973) Problems in the diagnosis and treatment of the sore throat syndrome. *Pediatrics Digest*, **15**, 37–44.

Wannamaker, L. W. (1972) Perplexity and precision in the diagnosis of streptococcal pharyngitis. *American Journal of Diseases of Children*, **124**, 352–358.

9

Infections of the cardiovascular system

Defences against infection
Portals of entry to the bloodstream are the skin, mucosae, the genitourinary, respiratory and intestinal tracts and each has its own particular set of defences against infection (see appropriate chapters). In the bloodstream itself the defence mechanisms include the neutrophil polymorphs and macrophages from the liver, spleen, lung and marrow as well as circulating antibodies.

The effectiveness of such defence mechanisms may be upset by several factors: (1) disturbance of the normal protective flora of the respiratory, intestinal and genital tracts by the administration of broad-spectrum antibiotics; (2) variations in the immune state of the host due to diabetes, steroid therapy, immunosuppression, immune deficiency diseases, blood dyscrasias and other malignancies; (3) the ability of some organisms such as *Salmonella typhi*, *Brucella* spp and *Mycobacterium tuberculosis* to survive and multiply within macrophages.

Potential pathogens. (see Fig. 9.1)

Bacteriaemia and septicaemia (see Ch. 2)

Organisms isolated from blood
The commonest isolates of clinical significance are *Staphylococcus aureus* and Gram-negative bacilli, including *Escherichia coli*, *Proteus*, *Pseudomonas*, *Klebsiella*, *Salmonella*, *Haemophilus*, *Bacteroides* and *Brucella* spp. *Streptococci*, particularly the viridans streptococci, *Streptococcus pneumoniae* and *Streptococcus faecalis* are also common isolates; neisseriae, clostridia, anaerobic cocci and *Staphylococcus albus* are less commonly found.

Predisposing factors
Peripheral sources include injury to the skin, for example surgical wounds, intravenous tubes, injection sites, burns and graft infections.

Central sources include therapeutic trauma such as sigmoidoscopy

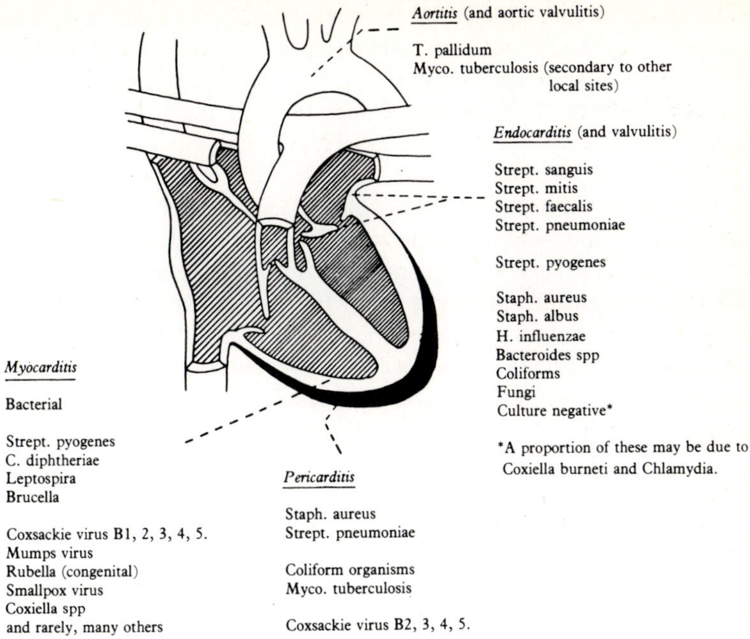

Fig. 9.1 Potential pathogens of the cardiovascular system

or even enemas, jejunal biopsy, catheterisation of the bladder, dilatation of the urethra and dental extraction. Collections of pus under pressure and infected tumours are also potential sources. In the patient receiving immunosuppressive drugs, cytotoxic drugs or corticosteroids, the immune mechanisms are less able to cope with invading organisms and organisms of lesser pathogenicity can produce septicaemia. Also, in the neonate with a congenital deformity the chances of septicaemia are high.

Infective endocarditis

Bacterial aetiology
Streptococcus sanguis, *Streptococcus mitis* and *Streptococcus faecalis* are most frequently involved, but also staphylococci, *Haemophilus influenzae*, *Bacteroides* spp, coliform organisms and anaerobic cocci. Rare non-bacterial causes are *Coxiella burneti* (Q fever) and *Chlamydia* (psittacosis agent). Fungal endocarditis may occur after the insertion of a prosthetic valve.

Pathogenesis and epidemiology
Patients at risk are those who have any pathology of the endocardium.

This includes congenital valve deformities, valve prostheses, suture material in the endocardium, atheroma of the valve, septal defects and, most commonly, damage to the valve from pre-existing rheumatic fever. Massive mixed infections of normal valves may occur in drug addicts who 'mainline'. Hypersensitivity may play a role in some cases. Minute platelet thrombi adhere to the roughened endothelium and in patients with a bacteriaemia bacteria may grow in the thrombi and produce fragile vegetations from which emboli can break off. The vegetations consist of fibrin and platelets and the bacteria are centrally placed in these. Fibrosis can occur in the valve and this surrounds and protects the bacteria even more extensively.

Acute and subacute forms can occur; pyogenic organisms are more common in the acute form. Over the years the major change in the pathogenesis has been a reduction in the number of cases caused by the viridans group of streptococci and an increase in those caused by the enterococci and staphylococci. Also, whereas the age group commonly involved was up to and around thirty years of age, nowadays infective endocarditis is becoming more and more a disease of the elderly and in these a previous history of rheumatic fever is still very common.

Laboratory examination

This is one of the many infections where close collaboration between ward and laboratory is vital in diagnosis and in the control of antimicrobial chemotherapy. Blood culture is the main diagnostic procedure. The mortality rate in blood culture-negative endocarditis exceeds that of cases where an organism has been identified.

Blood culture

Bacteria can be isolated from first cultures in more than 80 per cent of patients with infective endocarditis and bacteriaemia is often more persistent that intermittent. Many media can be used for culture of blood, such as cooked meat broth, brain heart infusion and thiol broth. It is important to subculture on to solid media and incubate both aerobically and anaerobically.

(See Ch. 4 for points to note in taking blood for culture).

Culture-negative endocarditis

Several reasons are suggested for this:

1. Chemotherapy has been started.
2. Bacteriaemia is intermittent and inadequate numbers of specimens have been taken.

3. Organisms may be fastidious or slow growers like *Bacteroides* spp; these require proper media and an adequate period of incubation. Nutritionally-variant strains, for example pyridoxine-dependent *Streptococcus mitis*, may be the causative agents and these will not grow on standard media.
4. Rickettsiae or chlamydiae may be involved; serological tests will clarify.
5. Occasionally organisms that may be reported as 'contaminants', for example *Staphylococcus albus*, may be the causative organisms.

Prophylaxis of infective endocarditis

This means antibiotic cover for susceptible persons during dental extractions, urinary tract and intestinal procedures and cardiac surgery.

For dental extraction susceptible persons should be given penicillin, preferably by *injection*, about 30 minutes before extraction. Penicillin with streptomycin or gentamicin may be given if culture of saliva has revealed penicillin-resistant viridans streptococci and patients with prosthetic valves should be given such a combination when undergoing dental treatment. Oral penicillin may be used if injections are refused or difficult to arrange and oral erythromycin may be substituted in penicillin-hypersensitive patients, started one hour before extraction, and, as with oral penicillin, continued for 24 hours.

Penicillin with streptomycin or gentamicin, or ampicillin with gentamicin are very suitable combinations in those undergoing urinary or intestinal tract manipulations because of the effect against *Streptococcus faecalis*.

In those about to undergo cardiac surgery a combination of benzyl penicillin or flucloxacillin and an aminoglycoside such as gentamicin will be effective against most relevant pathogenic bacteria.

Treatment

Laboratory monitoring of therapy is crucial and measurement of the MIC and MBC of antibiotics for the isolated organisms is required, particularly to ensure that serum levels are adequate to penetrate the valves and kill the bacteria. Doses have often to be very high to ensure this. It is essential that parenteral antibiotics are used at least for the first two weeks of treatment. There are reports of high levels of resistance to streptomycin in some strains of *Streptococcus faecalis*. Combined therapy may be more effective for all viridans streptococci as well as for the enterococci, for example a penicillin and an aminoglycoside; ampicillin or amoxycillin may be preferable to benzyl penicillin and in most cases gentamicin is the best choice of aminoglycoside. In all cases treatment must be continued for at least six weeks. In *Coxiella burneti* infection surgical excision of the valve is usually required with long term treatment with tetracyclines or clindamycin.

Rheumatic fever (RF)

Bacterial aetiology
Streptococcus pyogenes.

Pathogenesis and epidemiology
Two main theories have been proposed to explain the occurrence of this non-suppurative streptococcal complication: (1) that the initiation of the chronic lesions in the heart is due to the effect of some of the diffusible products of *Streptococcus pyogenes,* such as streptolysins O and S and proteinase; and (2) *the more accepted theory,* that immunological phenomena such as immune-complex disease, cross-reactive immunity or delayed hypersensitivity develop in certain persons who become sensitised to one or more streptococcal products. An immunological relationship exists between streptococcal antigens and human myocardial tissue and one such antigen responsible for cross-reactivity is localised in the cell wall and is associated with the M-protein. It is probable that several cross-reactive antigen-antibody systems occur between the streptococcus and heart tissue, and according to the currently-accepted theory cross-reactive antibody occurs to heart valves as well as to heart muscle, group-specific polysaccharide antigen of *Streptococcus pyogenes* having been found to cross-react with the structural glycoprotein of both human and bovine valves. Specific host factors have not been excluded in the pathogenesis of this disease. As well as the above examples of the connection between *Streptococcus pyogenes* and RF there is other evidence to associate the two, namely *clinical, bacteriological, epidemiological, serological* and *chemoprophylactic.*

Clinical
Physicians in an earlier era observed the common occurrence of RF a few weeks after an attack of scarlet fever and on many occasions patients admit to having had a sore throat several weeks before the onset of RF.

Bacteriological
Streptococcus pyogenes can often be isolated from the throat of RF patients.

Epidemiological

Altitude, humidity and other physical factors were all thought to have a role in the production of RF but it would now appear that RF can occur anywhere in the world. In general, rates increase when the streptococcal carriage rate increases and in the United Kingdom the age group which has the highest incidence of RF (seven to nine) is also that which has the highest incidence of streptococcal sore throat.

Serological

RF does not occur in the absence of immunological evidence of streptococcal infection. The first antibody to be measured was antistreptolysin O (ASO); titres become detectable in the second week after the onset of infection, are maximal by the sixth week and thereafter decrease. Other antibody levels can now be measured, such as antihyaluronidase (ASH), antistreptokinase (ASK), antideoxyribonuclease B (Anti DNAse B) and antinicotinamide adenine dinucleotidase (anti NADase). Most laboratories perform only the ASO and sometimes the anti DNAse B tests.

Chemoprophylaxis

There is proof that penicillin prophylaxis after a primary attack of RF will reduce substantially the risk of a second attack, by preventing further streptococcal infection of the throat.

Laboratory diagnosis

Throat swabs may or may not yield growth of *Streptococcus pyogenes* and so the most important investigations are serological. Two samples of serum must be assayed to check for a rising titre of antibody to *Streptococcus pyogenes* because a single estimation does not indicate whether a raised level of antibody pertains to a current infection or to one contracted several weeks or months previously.

Prophylaxis

The incidence of *primary attacks* is less than 1 per cent in the United Kingdom. To prevent these is virtually impossible. Penicillin treatment of streptococcal sore throat has been said to be of value in prevention but there is a great deal of evidence to show that this plays little part. For example, the incidence of RF in the United Kingdom had greatly decreased before the advent of antibiotics and, also, only a fraction of the population with streptococcal infection is treated with antibiotics because infection may be subclinical. In addition, the majority of persons with streptococcal sore throat tend not to visit their doctor for treatment. Prevention of second or subsequent attacks of RF is quite a different matter because the person who has had a primary attack of RF is prone to further attacks and daily prophylaxis using oral penicillin, or erythromycin in cases of hypersensitivity to penicillin, undoubtedly has proved of great benefit to these children.

Treatment

Benzyl or phenoxymethyl penicillin are the drugs of choice in non-hypersensitive patients in order to eliminate streptococci. Erythromycin is also useful.

Acute pericarditis

The most common causes of pericarditis are viruses (notably Coxsackie B and influenzae) and *Mycoplasma pneumoniae*. In general myocarditis and pericarditis occur together as an acute illness in young people. Bacterial causes are not common but *Staphylococcus aureus*, pneumococci and neisseriae may be involved either by direct spread from intrathoracic infection or as a complication of septicaemia. *Mycobacterium tuberculosis* may very occasionally be associated with the condition. Pericarditis is also a component of the rheumatic carditis syndrome.

FURTHER READING

Cruickshank, R. & Glynn, A. A. (1959) *Rheumatic Fever: Epidemiology and Prevention*. Oxford: Blackwell Scientific Publications.

Hayward, G. W. (1973) Infective endocarditis: a changing disease. *British Medical Journal*, **2**, 706–709; 764–766.

Haverkorn, M. J. (1974) *Streptococcal Disease and the Community*. Amsterdam: Excerpta Medica.

Munro, J. F., Duncan, L. J. P., & Durie, T. B. M. (1967) A clinical evaluation of blood cultures. *British Journal of Clinical Practice*, **21**, 71–74.

Uhr, J. W. (1964) *The Streptococcus, Rheumatic Fever and Glomerulonephritis*. Baltimore: Williams and Wilkins.

Wannamaker, L. W. & Matsen, J. M. (1972) *Streptococci and Streptococcal Diseases*. London: Academic Press.

Watt, B. (1978) Streptococcal endocarditis: a penicillin alone or a penicillin with an aminoglycoside? *Journal of Antimicrobial Chemotherapy*, **4**, 107–109.

10

Infections of the gastrointestinal tract

Normal flora

The stomach and upper small intestine in both adults and children is generally sterile in Europeans, although in certain Eastern races, due presumably to different dietary habits, streptococci and lactobacilli may be present; in general diet has a major effect on faecal flora. Once the ileum is reached, a typical Gram-negative bacillary flora is seen, composed mainly of *Escherichia coli.* The large intestine has a dense, varied flora the composition of which is influenced by the distribution and composition of the intestinal contents, local defence mechanisms, physiology of the host and diet. The organisms include *Escherichia coli, Streptococcus faecalis, Bacteroides* spp, *Lactobacillus* spp, *Clostridium* spp, anaerobic cocci, *Bifidobacterium* spp, *Klebsiella* spp, *Proteus* spp and *Pseudomonas* spp.

Defences against infection (see Table 10.1)

Table 10.1 Defences against infection in the alimentary tract

Dietary factors
Low pH of gastric juice
Lysozyme
Complement
Lactoferrin
Lymphokines
Intact normal flora
Local humoral mucosal antibody (secretory IgA)
IgG
Local cell-mediated mucosal antibody

Potential pathogens (see Fig. 10.1)

Cholera

Bacterial aetiology

Two vibrios, the classical *Vibrio cholerae* and the *El Tor* biotype cause cholera but other vibrios such as *Vibrio parahaemolyticus* can cause an

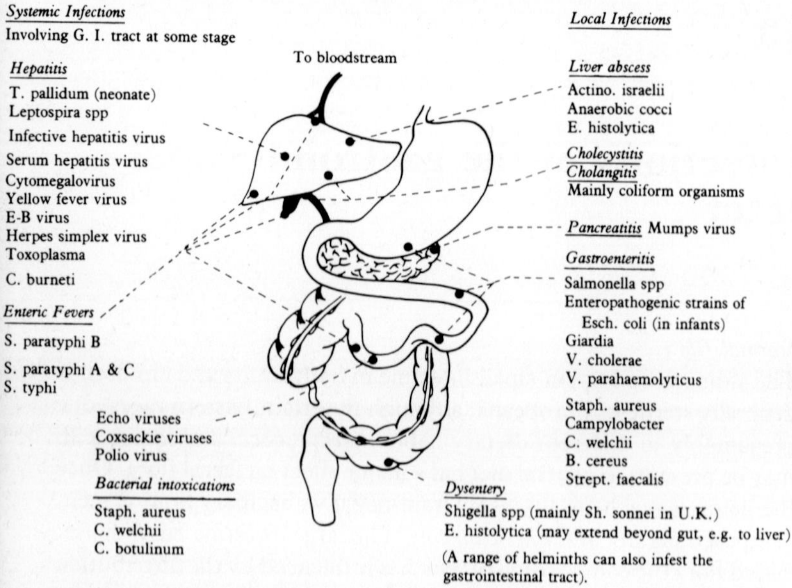

Fig. 10.1 Potential pathogens of the gastrointestinal tract

acute form of food poisoning. The two pathogenic biotypes can each be divided into two serological subtypes called *Inaba* and *Ogawa*.

Pathogenesis and epidemiology

Vibrios are ingested in food and water and surviving the acid barrier of the gastric juice begin to multiply in the intestinal contents, becoming attached to the epithelial cells of the small intestine. As they multiply in the lumen they produce a powerful enterotoxin whose action promotes increased outpouring of water and electrolytes into the intestine. There is no inflammatory reaction of the mucosa nor invasion of the intestinal wall. Lymph glands and blood are not affected. Effects of the disease such as severe dehydration are due to the massive outpouring of water and electrolytes. The resulting 'rice water' stools contain much mucus.

Cholera is highly communicable, transmitted from person to person via contaminated water or uncooked foods. During non-epidemic periods in endemic areas there is a high ratio of symptomless carriers to clinical cases particularly with the *El Tor* biotype, although explosive epidemics occur if a vehicle such as food or water is infected.

Laboratory diagnosis

A specimen of stool is examined for vibrios. In urgent cases a *vibrio immobilisation test* can be done under dark-field microscopy using specific antisera but it is most important to culture the organism by inoculation onto selective media such as bile-salt containing agar, and into a tube of alkaline peptone to encourage growth of vibrios should their numbers be small. Precise identification including biotyping and serotyping depends on further biochemical, serological and phage-sensitivity tests.

Prophylaxis
This includes isolation, treatment of infectious cases, surveillance of contacts and enforcement of proper community and group standards of hygiene. Prophylactic immunisation is not recommended because the available vaccines produce immunity that does not last longer than a few months.

Treatment
The most important treatment is to restore the vast loss of fluids and electrolytes. Later tetracyclines may be given to shorten the illness and reduce fluid requirements.

Dysentery

Bacterial aetiology
The genus *Shigella* contains four groups named *Shigella dysenteriae, flexneri, boydii* and *sonnei*. Each group is subdivided into various serotypes except *Shigella sonnei* which is serologically homogeneous.

Pathogenesis and epidemiology
Bacillary dysentery occurs by ingestion of the organisms. The bacilli attach themselves to the epithelial cells of the mucosal villi, enter these cells, multiply within them and spread into adjacent cells. The infected cells are killed and an inflammatory reaction results in the submucosa and lamina propria with resulting necrosis and ulceration of the epithelium. Invasion of the deeper layers does not generally take place. Stools contain blood, pus and mucus. *Shigella dysenteriae* infection is usually imported and causes a particularly severe form of dysentery because of the production of a powerful enterotoxin, in addition to the lipopolysaccharide endotoxin formed by all *Shigella* species. *Shigella flexneri* and *Shigella boydii* cause a less severe illness and *Shigella sonnei* infection which is the most common in the United Kingdom may only produce a few loose stools with slight abdominal discomfort.

In the main bacillary dysentery is spread from hand to mouth. A case or carrier can contaminate his hands at toilet and further contaminate door handles, lavatory chains and hand towels if his personal hygiene is deficient. Subsequent handling of these by another person results in the transfer of the dysentery bacilli to the hands and possibly the mouth. Pre-school and primary school children are frequently involved in outbreaks of dysentery. Inadequate toilet facilities and the lack of attention to hand washing undoubtedly play a part in the spread of the disease. Occasionally outbreaks may be food- or water-borne.

Laboratory diagnosis

A stool sample should be examined; this is much more satisfactory than a rectal swab. The swab is plated on MacConkey media and selective media such as deoxycholate citrate agar (DCA). (Xylose lysine deoxycholate agar (XLD) may be used as an alternative to DCA.) A fluid medium such as selenite broth should also be inoculated. Non-lactose fermenting colonies are then subjected to biochemical tests, and identified serologically.

Prophylaxis

Attention to hygiene is very important, for example the use of paper towels or hot air blowers rather than roller towels in institutions and the installation of washbasin taps operated by foot instead of by hand. Prophylactic use of antibiotics is a worthless exercise.

Treatment

Antibiotics have little part to play in this disease and may indeed prolong the period of excretion of the bacilli. An exception is the treatment of *Shigella dysenteriae* infection for which cotrimoxazole, ampicillin and tetracyclines may be used.

Enteric fever

Bacterial aetiology

The term *enteric fever* includes typhoid and paratyphoid A, B and C infections and are caused by *Salmonella typhi* and *Salmonella paratyphi* respectively. Other serotypes of *Salmonella* do not cause enteric fever but *salmonellosis,* a form of food poisoning.

Pathogenesis and epidemiology

Table 10.2 shows the pathogenesis of enteric fever and it can be seen that bacteriaemia is the important feature of the illness; the bacilli are also present in large numbers in many organs. The pathogenicity of salmonellae appears to depend both on their ability to survive and grow inside macrophages and on the toxicity of their lipopolysaccharide *O antigen*. In addition, typhoid bacilli possess a glycolipid microcapsule called the *virulence* (*Vi*) antigen which protects the organism against phagocytosis and antibody.

The source of typhoid and paratyphoid infections is *man*, either as a case or carrier and spread can be via water, food, or the faecal-oral routes. The most common cause of enteric fever in the United Kingdom is *Salmonella paratyphi B*.

After an attack of enteric fever the organisms may persist in the gall bladder and are excreted intermittently in the faeces.

Table 10.2 Pathogenesis of enteric fever

Salmonella typhi

↓

Intestine

↓

Mesenteric lymph nodes

↓

Bloodstream (via thoracic duct)

↓ Primary bacteriaemia (First 7–10 days of incubation period)

Liver

Spleen

Gallbladder → intestine → faeces

Kidney

Bone marrow

↓ Secondary bacteriaemia (Symptoms and signs of clinical illness)

Several organs (e.g. kidney → urine)
(gall bladder → intestine → faeces)

Laboratory diagnosis

Specimens required for diagnosis vary according to the stage of the infection. During the first seven to ten days blood culture is the examination of choice and in the second and third weeks stool cultures are usually positive; urine cultures may also be positive at this stage. A test for agglutinating antibody in serum, the Widal reaction, can be done in the second or third weeks but is of limited value as false positive results are common. Blood, stool and urine cultures are the most important tests and should be done repeatedly.

Blood cultures are subcultured to blood agar plates and coliform-type colonies are tested for their sugar fermentation reactions. Non-lactose fermenting colonies are subjected to further biochemical and serological tests. Stools and urine are subcultured on MacConkey agar and DCA; non-lactose fermenting colonies are picked for further testing.

Prophylaxis

Safer water supplies, adequate sewage disposal and attention to personal hygiene are of great importance. Bacteriological surveillance of workers in the food industry is essential. Immunisation is commonly practised with TAB vaccine which consists of heat-killed *Salmonella typhi* and *Salmonella paratyphi* A and B organisms preserved in phenol.

Treatment

Chloramphenicol, ampicillin and cotrimoxazole are useful drugs both in the treatment of acute typhoid fever, and of the carrier state. Cholecystectomy is often required when there is chronic gall bladder carriage.

Food poisoning

Bacterial aetiology

In the United Kingdom *Salmonella* spp (particularly *typhimurium*) and *Campylobacter* spp account for most cases. Other organisms implicated, in order of frequency, are *Clostridium welchii*, *Staphylococcus aureus*, *Escherichia coli* and *Bacillus cereus*. Rarely *Vibrio parahaemolyticus* and *Streptococcus faecalis* may be involved.

Pathogenesis and epidemiology

This is an acute form of gastroenteritis due to bacterial contamination of food or drink. There are two main types: (1) The *infective type* and (2) the *toxic type*.

(1) *Infective type*: Ingestion of food contaminated with salmonellae leads to this type of food poisoning. The infecting organisms multiply in the food and later in the intestine of the victim. Many different species of *Salmonella* may be responsible for this type of infection,

including *Salmonella typhimurium, heidelberg, enteritidis, dublin* and *thompson*. The 12–48 hour incubation period is longer than in toxic food poisoning and is followed by pyrexia and diarrhoea of one or two days' duration. Vomiting is not usually severe. Cold meats, poultry, sausages and occasionally eggs are common sources of salmonellae. Infection may be direct from an infected carcase or acquired from cases and carriers among food handlers if there is general lack of hygiene, inadequate cooking of foods and inadequate thawing of foods, particularly poultry, before cooking.

(2) *Toxic type*: This is most commonly produced by *Staphylococcus aureus* and *Clostridium welchii*, both of which produce an enterotoxin. Staphylococcal food poisoning causes nausea, vomiting and often prostration with some diarrhoea within one to six hours of ingesting the contaminated food containing the pre-formed heat-stable toxin. Foods commonly incriminated include cream cakes, trifles, meat paste, pies and ham. The usual sources of staphylococci are the upper respiratory tract, particularly the nose, and septic lesions on the skin of food handlers. In *Clostridium welchii* food poisoning, abdominal cramps followed by diarrhoea occur around 8–12 hours after ingestion of contaminated food. Fever and vomiting are rare. *Clostridium welchii* is a sporing organism that can withstand the heat of cooking and multiply freely in conditions where food is allowed to cool slowly or where it is gently reheated before serving. Foods commonly associated are bulk meat dishes such as stews. The source of organisms may be either the meat itself or the intestine of the food handler. A dose of 10^7–10^8 organisms is required to initiate infection and the symptoms of infection are due to an enterotoxin which is produced in the intestine, and not preformed in the food. Enterotoxin production is associated with sporulation of the organisms. In general, food poisoning is far more common than it should be and is related to the many commercially-prepared foodstuffs and catered meals. The summer is the commonest season for outbreaks because of high ambient temperatures and lack of refrigeration of prepared foods, allowing multiplication of organisms.

Laboratory diagnosis

Specimens of vomit, faeces and suspected foods should be sent for analysis and bacterial culture. Salmonellae when identified may be phage-typed and *Clostridium welchii* isolates should be serotyped.

Prophylaxis

Meat inspection, routine medical inspection of food handlers and education in matters of hygiene for all food handlers should be encouraged. Hygienic premises, adequate cooking and use of refrigeration are essential. Raw and cooked meats must be kept separately.

Treatment

Fluid balance, particularly in the elderly and the very young, must be maintained. The use of antibiotics is not recommended in most cases as they do not shorten the duration of the diarrhoea and do not eliminate the causal organisms.

The following are less common causes of food poisoning in the United Kingdom:

Bacillus cereus. This is associated with rice, and symptoms are probably due to preformed enterotoxin. Two clinical types are described: (1) staphylococcal-like, of rapid onset and with vomiting as the main feature, and (2) clostridial-like, with a longer incubation period and with diarrhoea and abdominal pain.

Vibrio parahaemolyticus. The organism producing this type of food poisoning is a marine vibrio associated with shellfish. The organism multiplies in the intestine and may produce a cholera-like enterotoxin. Patients usually suffer from vomiting, diarrhoea and abdominal pain.

Infantile gastroenteritis

Bacterial aetiology

Enteropathogenic strains of *Escherichia coli* that are responsible for infantile gastroenteritis are limited to a small number of 'O' serotypes with an associated B-type K antigen, for example 026,B6; 055,B5 and 0111,B4.

Pathogenesis and epidemiology

An enterotoxin similar to cholera exotoxin in its mode of action is produced; some strains may be locally invasive like shigellae or penetrate more deeply like salmonellae. In infants the disease is sometimes known as *cholera infantum* and causes a massive loss of fluid from the small intestine, often resulting in peripheral circulatory failure.

Outbreaks occur in infant nurseries and day nurseries as well as in the normal population and most patients are under 18 months of age. There is a higher incidence in artifically-fed babies.

Immunity in older children and adults may be due to acquired local immunity in the intestine.

Laboratory diagnosis

Faeces are plated on blood agar and MacConkey agar. Agglutination tests are performed on *Escherichia coli* isolated using sera containing antibodies to O and B antigens.

Prophylaxis

Attention to personal and environmental hygiene, proper nutrition and breast feeding of babies will lessen the incidence of the disease.

Treatment

Rehydration and restoration of the electrolyte balance is vital. Antibiotic chemotherapy may be of benefit in mild cases but cannot act quickly enough in the acute stages.

Abscesses

Subphrenic abscess

Bacterial aetiology. *Staphylococcus aureus* and, in particular, organisms found in the intestinal flora such as coliform organisms and *Streptococcus faecalis*, are involved. The flora is commonly mixed.

Pathogenesis. The peritoneum in this area is arranged in a complicated fashion with the result that there are seven spaces in which pus may collect, three on either side of the body and one in the midline. A subphrenic abscess can be caused as a sequel to a perforated peptic ulcer, trauma, appendicitis and leakage after gall bladder and stomach operations. Empyema may be associated.

Laboratory diagnosis. Aspiration of the pus is the best way to obtain a specimen for bacterial diagnosis; pus is Gram-stained and cultured aerobically and anaerobically. Blood cultures should be taken.

Treatment. This is surgical drainage with or without antibiotic therapy.

Pelvic abscess

Bacterial aetiology. This is much the same as for subphrenic abscess. Organisms from the faecal or vaginal flora including anaerobes are commonly involved.

Pathogenesis. This can be a complication of appendicitis or salpingitis, and there may be an associated peritonitis.

Laboratory diagnosis and treatment. As for subphrenic abscess; surgical drainage is essential.

Peritonitis

Bacterial aetiology

This is variable depending on the source of infection and includes normal intestinal bacteria such as coliform organisms, *Streptococcus faecalis*, anaerobic cocci and *Bacteroides* spp. Frequently more than one organism is isolated.

Pathogenesis

Infection can be *direct* or *septicaemic*. *Direct* infection originates from perforation of an area of the intestine from trauma or following surgery. The appendix, gall bladder, fallopian tubes and damaged intestine, for example from a carcinoma, are common sources. Peritonitis may remain *localised* when the cause is an inflamed appendix or become *generalised* when caused by perforation of a peptic ulcer.

Laboratory diagnosis

Any exudate or pus that can be obtained from drainage should be examined microscopically and cultured aerobically and anaerobically. Bacteriaemia frequently occurs in conjunction with peritonitis and blood cultures must be taken.

Treatment

Surgical treatment is frequently essential and antibiotics, often in combinations, are urgently required. If treatment has to be blind the possibility of the involvement of anaerobic organisms must be considered. A penicillin or clindamycin may be administered along with an aminoglycoside such as gentamicin. Metronidazole is effective against *Bacteroides* spp.

Bacteria and malignant disease

The nature of the diet affects the composition of the intestinal flora and determines the substrates available for bacterial metabolism and a relationship between diet and malignant disease of the intestine has been postulated. The incidence of malignant disease, in particular cancer of the colon, has been shown to correlate strongly with the amount of dietary fat and animal protein and not at all with dietary fibre. It is thought that carcinogenic substances may be produced by the action of bacteria on certain dietary components and intestinal secretions.

FURTHER READING

Christie, A. B. (1974) *Infectious Diseases: Epidemiology and Clinical Practice.* Edinburgh: Churchill Livingstone.

Collee, J. G. (1974) Bacterial challenges in food. *Postgraduate Medical Journal*, **50**, 636–43.

Collee, J. G. (1976) *Applied Medical Microbiology.* Oxford: Blackwell Scientific Publications.

Geddes, A. M. (1973); Enteric fever, salmonellosis and food poisoning. *British Medical Journal*, **1**, 98–100.

Hendrickse, R. G. (1972) Dysentery including amoebiasis. *British Medical Journal*, **1**, 669–672.

Hobbs, B. C. (1968) *Food Poisoning and Food Hygiene.* London: Arnold.

Lowbury, E. J. L., Ayliffe, G. A. J., Geddes, A. M. & Williams, J. O. (1975) *Control of Hospital Infection: A Practical Handbook.* London: Chapman and Hall.

11

Infections of the urinary tract

Normal flora of the urethra
Several species of organisms may be found as commensals in the distal urethra and most of these are derived from faecal flora. Organisms include *Escherichia coli*, *Proteus* spp, *Klebsiella* spp, *Pseudomonas* spp, various other coliform organisms, staphylococci, streptococci, lactobacilli, mycoplasmas and ureaplasmas.

Defences against infection
Bladder urine is normally sterile because of hydrokinetic and mucosal factors. Hydrokinetic aspects include the periodic voiding of urine, the constant dilution of residual urine in the bladder by inflow from the kidneys and the completeness of emptying of the bladder. The bacteriocidal mechanisms in the bladder mucosa cause a rapid clearing of bacteria from the mucosa, the mechanism of which is unclear but may be immunological. Local antibody, complement and lysozyme may also be protective. Prostatic secretions and periurethral gland secretions also possess antibacterial factors.

Potential pathogens (see Fig. 11.1)

Glomerulonephritis

Aetiology
Poststreptococcal glomerulonephritis is a common type of acute nephritis but there may be other aetiological agents including viruses. In comparison with rheumatic fever which can be caused by a large variety of types of *Streptococcus pyogenes*, acute glomerulonephritis (AGN) is produced by a very much narrower range of serotypes.

Pathogenesis and epidemiology
Human AGN relates both to *infection* and *immunity*; theories as to its production include the following:

Soluble-complex induced. Soluble complexes, or toxic complexes, circulate in the body having escaped the action of the phagocytes. The

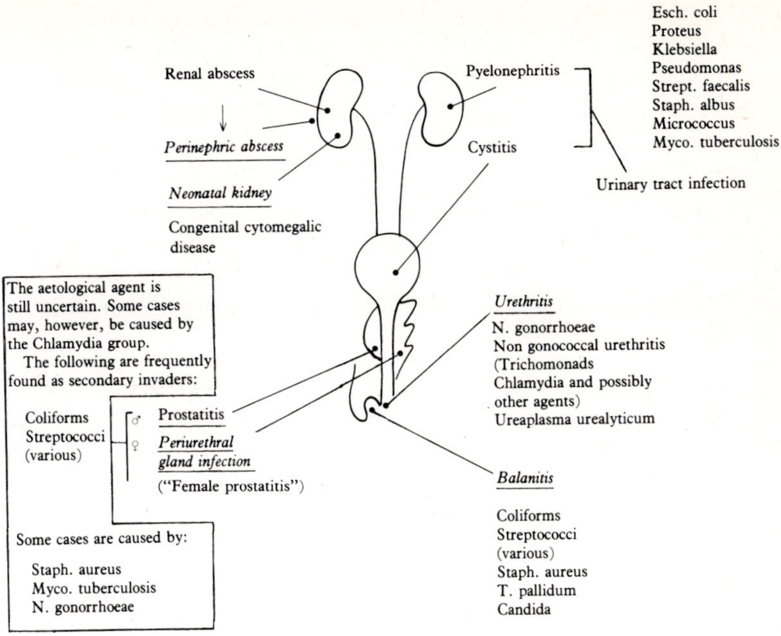

Fig. 11.1 Potential pathogens of the urinary system

complexes which consist of antigen, antibody and complement are filtered off in the glomerulus, from which they are generally removed after several weeks. Antigen involved is quite unrelated to the kidney.

Antikidney antibody. (Anti-glomerular-basement-membrane antibody). Normal persons release glomerular-basement-membrane-reacting fragments in both plasma and urine and at times these may become immunogenic.

Pathogenetic mechanisms may also relate to cross reactions between streptococcal membrane antigens and other human membrane antigens, including the glomerular-basement-membrane.

Whichever of the theories is correct— and all may be involved from time to time— the events that follow the combination of antigen and antibody in the kidney are the same, namely *activation of complement* and *coagulation*. The main cause of injury to the glomerulus is caused by activation of complement with the concomitant attraction of leucocytes and immune adherence with release of enzymes from the leucocytes. Complement components, particularly C3, are reduced in AGN. Complement also initiates *coagulation* which leads to local tissue damage through microthrombosis and inflammation. Although the above events are all potentially reversible the healing processes quite often produce scarring.

The role of both skin and throat infections in the development of

AGN is now firmly established, although there are clear differences in the epidemiology. For example, AGN following streptococcal throat infection occurs at the colder times of the year and mostly in children, whereas AGN following infected skin lesions (*pyoderma*) such as impetigo occurs in all age groups in the hot humid weather, notably in Alabama and the West Indies, where the Hippelates fly is an important vector of streptococci. The nephritogenic serotypes are also different. AGN following throat infection can be caused by M-types 12, 1, 25, 4 and 3, whereas AGN following pyoderma involves M-types 49 and 52, 53, 54; 55, 57, 58; 59, 60, 61. Recurrences of AGN are rare.

Laboratory diagnosis

Although beta-haemolytic streptococci may be isolated from the throat and skin, serological tests are generally more helpful. Immune responses vary depending on whether the source of infection is the throat or skin. For example, the *antistreptolysin O* (ASO) estimation is reliable in the throat form but unreliable in pyoderma-associated AGN, whereas the *anti-deoxyribonuclease B* (*anti-DNAse B*) titre is raised more frequently and to a greater degree in pyoderma-associated AGN.

Prophylaxis

By treating skin lesions AGN may be prevented, but treatment of throat infections has little effect.

Treatment

Antibiotics are ineffective in established AGN.

Urinary tract infection (UTI)

Bacterial aetiology

Escherichia coli is responsible for the greatest number of cases but many other bacteria are involved including *Streptococcus faecalis*, *Proteus* spp, *Pseudomonas aeruginosa*, *Micrococcus* group 3, *Klebsiella* spp and *Staphylococcus albus*.

Pathogenesis and epidemiology

Although terms such as cystitis and pyelonephritis are used, UTI is not always confined to one particular anatomical site and the urinary tract should therefore be considered as a whole. Attempts to localise UTI clinically may be difficult.

Frequency and *dysuria* are common symptoms, especially in females, of all ages, but a positive urine culture is found in only a proportion of cases. Culture-negative and culture-positive cases are clinically indistinguishable. Infection generally spreads directly from the perineum, aided in females by the short distance between urethra and anus, the interposition of the vaginal introitus and the shortness of the urethra. Haematogenous spread is rare. Various factors contribute to this type of infection such as poor personal hygiene, menstruation, sexual intercourse, pregnancy and, in older women, gynaecological problems such as prolapse and vaginitis. Incomplete emptying of the bladder due to mechanical obstruction or neurological defects may also produce a source of residual urine that can become infected.

Asymptomatic bacteriuria

Transient symptomless bacteriuria is common in the female and is usually a benign condition with spontaneous resolution, although in the pregnant woman or in childhood there can be progressive renal disease and damage. If there are congenital abnormalities in the urinary tract or some form of obstruction bacteriuria may persist and produce symptoms.

Renal infection may follow infection of an obstructed urinary tract, for example due to the presence of calculi. Vesicoureteric reflux is reasonably common particularly in children and is of paramount importance in the production of renal damage; the reflux can carry organisms into the substance of the kidney and it is also a source of residual urine in the bladder. In addition it may produce damage by back pressure, resulting ultimately in chronic pyelonephritis; renal scarring is not common after infection in the absence of reflux. The renal medulla is very susceptible to infections; it is the site of ammonia production which has a powerful anti-complementary effect.

Laboratory diagnosis

Bacteriological examination of the urine is essential for confirmation of the diagnosis, control of chemotherapy and assessment of the results of treatment.

The diagnosis of urinary tract infection relies principally on the demonstration of significant bacteriuria by quantitative culture of a fresh or refrigerated midstream specimen of urine (MSSU). A viable count of above 10^5 organisms of a single bacterial species per ml of urine indicates a *true infection* (significant bacteriuria); between 10^4 and 10^5 organisms per ml is of *doubtful significance* and may indicate either infection or heavy contamination (only a few specimens fall into this 'doubtful' group); 10^4 organisms per ml are sometimes found in the absence of infection and also when a patient is on antibiotic therapy.

Specimen collection

Proper collection of specimens is essential and because urine is a good culture medium it is important that specimens reach the laboratory with the minimum of delay, or that they are refrigerated until despatched. The following specimens can be obtained:

Midstream specimen (MSSU) (see Ch. 4).

Suprapubic aspiration of bladder urine. If it is difficult to collect an MSSU, or previous findings have been equivocal, it may be worthwhile to consider suprapubic aspiration.

Urine specimens from infants. Bag specimens are unsatisfactory. A 'clean catch' specimen is adequate if the infant can be caught in the act, but suprapubic aspiration is a simple procedure and gives the most satisfactory and reliable results.

Catheter specimens of urine should be submitted only if the catheter is already *in situ*. The sample should be collected directly from the catheter and not from the collection bag.

Examination of MSSU

Microscopy. This is useful for detecting pus cells, epithelial cells, red blood cells and bacteria and should be performed on a *centrifuged* deposit. Both wet films and Gram-stained films may be examined.

Culture. Specimens are usually isolated on nutrient agar and MacConkey agar.

Quantitative culture. This is done using a well-mixed specimen by the method of Miles and Misra. It is a surface viable count, and gives accurate results, but as it is a time-consuming test it cannot be used routinely in a busy service laboratory.

Semiquantitative culture. This kind of culture provides useful information. There are three commonly used methods: (1) transfer of a fixed volume of undiluted urine to a suitable culture medium by a calibrated loop; (2) the blotting-paper strip method; (3) dip-slides.

The blotting-paper strip, of known area, is dipped in the urine then impressed on MacConkey agar. Colony counts within the area can then be related to numbers of organisms per ml.

Dip slides. (Plastic slides coated with CLED agar (Cystine lactose electrolyte-deficient) on one side and MacConkey agar on the other) can be obtained commercially. A slide is dipped into the freshly-passed urine; a semi-quantitative assessment of the viable count is obtained by comparing the density of growth on the media, after incubation, with the manufacturers' graded charts. Dip-slides avoid the problems of transporting specimens, particularly from General Practitioners' surgeries, and are useful in screening for significant bacteriuria in busy out-patient clinics, for example ante-natal clinics. The incubated slides should be examined in the bacteriology laboratory. (Interpretation of mixed cultures is difficult with dip slides).

Results of semi-quantitiative culture from fresh or refrigerated urine
The results may be reported as:

1. *No growth.*
2. *No significant growth* (less than 10^4 organisms per ml, or scanty mixed contaminants).
3. *Many mixed organisms* (indicating faecal contamination of the specimen).
4. *Approximately 10^4 organisms per ml, of doubtful significance.* (If composed of several bacterial species, for example *Staphylococcus albus*, lactobacilli or diphtheroid organisms, this probably represents contamination although the detection of 10^4 organisms per ml of a single species may occasionally be significant).
5. *A significant growth* (greater than 10^5 organisms per ml of a single species, or occasionally two species).

In acute infections the growth is usually of a single organism which in some 75 per cent of cases is *Escherichia coli*; in chronic infections the cultures may contain more than one organism and *Klebsiella*, *Proteus* and *Pseudomonas* species and *Streptococcus faecalis* (enterococci) are most common. A few infections are caused by micrococci and *Staphylococcus albus*.

Prophylaxis of UTI
This can be achieved by long-term administration of antibiotics usually in reduced dose to kill any organisms that enter the bladder from the gut, although the danger is an increase in the resistance of the intestinal flora. Where predisposing causes exist such as renal calculi or obstruction to the outflow of the bladder surgical intervention will be required.

Treatment
Asymptomatic infection needs no treatment except during pregnancy and possibly during childhood. *Symptomatic infection* demands adequate urinary concentration of antibacterial agents to which the organism is sensitive. Useful agents include cotrimoxazole, nitrofurantoin and nalidixic acid. Cephalosporins and ampicillin may be used but there are now many reports of high levels of resistance to ampicillin in *Escherichia coli* particularly in hospital practice. A problem is a high recurrence rate, either by relapse which indicates

failure of the initial treatment to eradicate the organism, or reinfection. In patients with indwelling catheters bladder washouts are useful.

Genito-urinary tuberculosis

Tuberculosis of the kidney is a consequence of invasion of the blood by *Mycobacterium tuberculosis*; early lesions occur first in the blood vessels surrounding the glomeruli. These microscopic foci expand, erode into the collecting system and hence into the pelvis, with downward spread to the bladder, and produce tuberculous cystitis. The epididymis and seminal vesicles may also become infected. Frequently routine culture of the urine is negative and in many of these cases a Gram-stained film shows pus cells without organisms. In cases of pyuria without bacteriuria tuberculosis must be considered.

Excretion of tubercle bacilli from the kidney is intermittent and because of this an MSSU is quite unsuitable for laboratory examination. *Instead, at least 100 ml of early morning urine (EMU)* should be sent to the laboratory, on three consecutive days. Ziehl-Neelsen films are examined on a spun deposit and culture is performed on Löwenstein-Jensen, modified Löwenstein-Jensen or sodium pyruvate media. Guinea-pig inoculation is a useful procedure in suspected renal tuberculosis.

Treatment

This must be continued for a period of nine months to two years, using modern anti-tuberculous drugs (see Ch. 8).

Perinephric abscess

This can arise: (1) by extension of an abscess in the cortex of a kidney; (2) by extension of an appendix abscess via periureteral lymphatics; (3) from the blood. Surgical drainage, with or without antibiotics, is the treatment of choice.

FURTHER READING

Asscher, A. W. (1974) Pathogenesis and management of urinary tract infection in women. *British Journal of Hospital Medicine*, **12**, 546–554.

Asscher, A. W. (1978) Management of frequency and dysuria. *British Medical Journal*, **1**, 1531–1533.

Cameron, J. S. (1972) Bright's disease today: the pathogenesis and treatment of glomerulonephritis. *British Medical Journal*, **4**, 87–90; 160–163; 217–220.

Dillon, H. C. (1970) Streptococcal skin infection and acute glomerulonephritis. *Postgraduate Medical Journal*, **46**, 641–652.

Duerden, B. I. & Moyes, A. (1976) Comparison of laboratory methods in the diagnosis of urinary tract infection. *Journal of Clinical Pathology*, **29**, 286–291.

Haverkorn, M. (1974) *Streptococcal Disease and the Community*. Amsterdam: Excerpta Medica.

O'Grady, F. & Brumfitt, W. (1968) *Urinary Tract Infection*. London: Oxford University Press.

Sleigh, J. D., Robertson, J. G. & Isdale, M. H. (1964) Asymptomatic bacteriuria in pregnancy. *Journal of Obstetrics and Gynaecology*, **71**, 74–81.

Uhr, J. W. (1964) *The Streptococcus, Rheumatic Fever and Glomerulonephritis*. Baltimore: Williams and Wilkins.

12

Infections of the genital tract

Normal flora of the vagina

The vagina is colonised very soon after birth. In considering the normal flora of the region it is important to remember the various ecological areas in and around the vagina, such as the periurethral glands, Bartholin's glands and the cervical canal. Organisms are not uniformly distributed throughout the female genital tract and some areas support growth of predominantly anaerobic flora whereas others support the growth of the more common aerobes. The biochemical properties of mucus may contribute to the numbers, types and location of bacteria in the female genital tract.

Many different species can be cultured from the vaginal area depending on the methods used for isolation and on the site sampled. In general there are several groups of organisms commonly present: lactobacilli, diphtheroids, group B streptococci, anaerobic cocci, coliform organisms, *Streptococcus faecalis, Staphylococcus albus, Bacteroides* spp and yeasts.

Several authors have postulated differences in the vaginal flora of the pregnant and non-pregnant woman but the differences are not constant. Sexual factors as well as physiological factors may play a more important role in determining numbers and species of organisms, and because it is not absolutely clear which organisms are pathogens in the vagina it is not strictly possible to describe what is normal flora.

Defences against infection in the female genital tract

The presence of glycogen in the vaginal mucosa, controlled by the secretion of oestrogens and progesterone and acted upon by lactobacilli (Doderlein's bacilli) to produce lactic acid and an environment of pH 5, is an important mechanism of protection in the vagina. This pertains to the newborn, whose hormones are derived from the mother, and to women in the reproductive age group. During childhood and after the menopause when oestrogen activity is absent glycogen is not deposited in the vaginal mucosa and the vaginal pH rises to between 6 and 7.

The flora of the vagina and of the periurethral area prevents colonisation by other species and an intact epithelium is also important in this.

Potential pathogens (see Fig. 12.1)

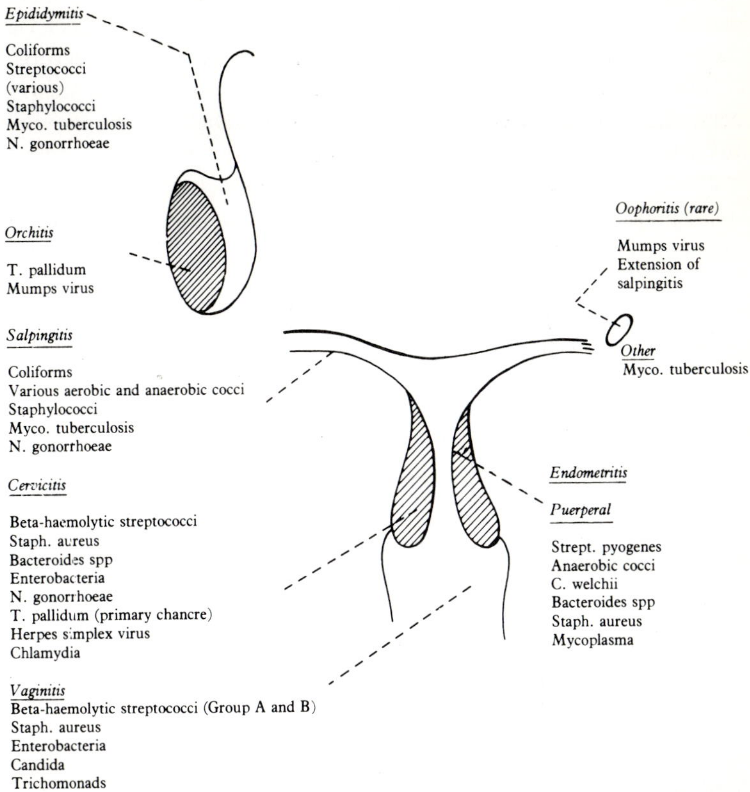

Fig. 12.1 Potential pathogens of the genital tract

Puerperal pyrexia

Puerperal pyrexia is defined in Scotland as a temperature of 38°C (100°F) sustained for 24 hours, or recurring within that period, during the 21 days after childbirth. In England and Wales 14 days are postulated. Sources of pyrexia are most commonly genital, breast, urinary or respiratory infection.

Puerperal sepsis (Childbed fever)

Bacterial aetiology

Many bacteria can produce infection in the postpartum uterus, most commonly *Staphylococcus aureus*, beta-haemolytic streptococci, anaerobic cocci, *Streptococcus faecalis*, *Bacteroides* spp and coliform organisms.

Pathogenesis and epidemiology

Infection can be endogenous or exogenous. Endogenous sources are the upper respiratory tract, skin and hair of the patient where there may be staphylococci and streptococci, and the alimentary tract via the perineum from where infection may be caused by the anaerobic cocci and enterobacteria. Exogenous sources are either similar sites in personnel looking after the patient, or environmental, and may be airborne, transferred by infected hands, or the result of careless instrumentation. Puerperal sepsis is basically a wound infection with consequent inflammatory reaction in the pelvic organs. Nowadays infection rarely spreads from the placental site to the tubes and ovaries because of antibiotic therapy.

Laboratory diagnosis

High vaginal swabs and particularly cervical swabs may be helpful but pus or discharge should be processed if obtainable. Care should be taken to ensure that sufficient media are used to facilitate isolation of the more fastidious organisms, particularly anaerobes. Blood must be taken for culture.

Treatment

This will depend on laboratory reports although it is often necessary to start treatment on an empirical basis until accurate information can be obtained. Combined therapy with a penicillin or aminoglycoside with metronidazole (as infection is often anaerobic) is generally effective.

Vulvitis

This is commonly caused by *Trichomonas vaginalis* and yeasts but may be caused occasionally by gonococci. *Vulvo-vaginitis* occurs in young girls often as the result of inadequate perineal hygiene but sometimes as a sequel to the presence of some foreign body in the vagina. Staphylococci and coliform organisms are often isolated and occasionally gonococci. *Bartholinitis,* acute infection of the gland and duct of Bartholin in the posterior third of the labia majora, may also be associated with gonococci, coliform organisms and anaerobic bacteria.

Vaginitis

In addition to trichomonal and yeast infection a non-specific form of vaginitis occurs from which staphylococci, streptococci (groups A and

B), coliform organisms and other intestinal organisms may be isolated; this may be associated with the use of pessaries, douches and tampons.

Cervicitis

Acute cervicitis may be *primary* as the result of injury, for example an accidental tear during childbirth, or *secondary* due to inflammatory lesions in the endometrium or vagina. Staphylococci, streptococci, coliform organisms, gonococci, *Bacteroides* spp, as well as trichomonads and yeasts, may be involved, and acute cervicitis may also occur in sexually transmitted diseases such as chancroid and lymphogranuloma venereum.

Endometritis

The myometrium and pelvic peritoneum may also be involved. This occurs most commonly following childbirth and abortions, and as the result of gonorrhoeal infection.

Salpingitis

Acute salpingitis may occur: (1) by upward spread of infection from the uterus along the mucosa of the tube, as in gonococcal infection; (2) from the pelvic cellular tissue to which infection has spread from the endometrium through the uterine wall, by veins and lymphatics. Here the tube is attacked from the periphery, infection proceeding from outside into the mucosa of the tube, as in post-abortal or puerperal salpingitis; (3) from the bowel as in appendicitis; and (4) by the bloodstream as in tuberculosis.

The ovaries are usually also involved (salpingo-oophoritis), the condition is commonly bilateral and there is frequently an associated pelvic peritonitis.

Pelvic cellulitis

This is generally combined with pelvic peritonitis. Infection is usually confined to the tissues of the pelvic floor. It may start in one broad ligament and spread to the other, in front of and behind the uterus, or may spread upwards via the cervix; occasionally salpingo-oophoritis may occur. Pelvic cellulitis follows injury to the upper vagina and cervix as the result of parturition, abortion, pelvic surgery and careless dilatation of the cervix; it may follow appendicitis, diverticulitis and infection of a bowel carcinoma. Abscess formation nowadays rarely occurs.

In all gynaecological infections adequate specimens are essential for helpful bacteriological reports. Blood cultures must be taken. When specimens cannot be obtained 'best-guess' antibiotic therapy may be required.

Urethritis

Neisseria gonorrhoeae, although most commonly involved in acute urethritis, can also cause *prostatitis. Non-specific urethritis* is produced in over 50 per cent of cases by *Chlamydia trachomatis.* Essential specimens for examination include a urethral swab and pus. *Balanitis* is associated with various organisms and a swab should be taken from inside the prepuce.

Epididymitis

Although infection may be confined to the epididymis, *epididymo-orchitis* may also occur.

Infection occurs via the vas and is usually secondary to infection of the urinary tract, prostate and seminal vesicles. It can also occur after prostatectomy and urethral instrumentation.

Gram-negative bacilli, particularly those associated with urinary tract infection, are frequently involved, and to a lesser extent staphylococci and gonococci. *Mycobacterium tuberculosis* and viruses, including mumps, are infrequent causes.

Culture of urine with consequent antimicrobial chemotherapy is essential.

Orchitis

This can occur either as an extention of epididymitis or via the bloodstream. In the latter viruses, particularly mumps and coxsackie, are commonly involved.

SEXUALLY-TRANSMITTED DISEASES

These are the most common communicable diseases after the common cold and their incidence increases yearly. Only a minority of patients suffer from the classical venereal diseases such as syphilis (*Treponema pallidum*), gonorrhoea (*Neisseria gonorrhoeae*), chancroid (*Haemophilus ducreyi*), lymphogranuloma venereum (*Chlamydia*), granuloma inguinale (*Donovania granulomatis*).

The majority of patients suffer from the following:

Non-specific urethritis (caused by *Chlamydia* in 50 per cent of cases)
Trichomoniasis (*Trichomonas vaginalis*)
Genital candidiasis (*Candida albicans*)

Warts (Papilloma virus)
Molluscum contagiosum (a pox virus)
Genital herpes simplex
Ectoparasite infestation (crab louse; scabies).

Chancroid

Haemophilus ducreyi produces a soft sore or chancroid, a venereal disease that may be confused with syphilis. Organisms can be identified in the exudate and pus from the genital sore; there are special nutritional requirements for their isolation.

Gonorrhoea

Bacterial aetiology

Neisseria gonorrhoeae (the gonococcus).

Pathogenesis and epidemiology

The gonococcus is a strictly human parasite and unlike the meningococcus is seldom found in carriers, although asymptomatic carriers do occur. The anterior urethra is affected in men and the anterior urethra and cervix in women and infection is generally limited to the mucosa, although spread in men can affect the prostate, seminal vesicles and epididymis. In women advanced infection may affect the uterus and fallopian tubes although the vaginal mucosa is rarely involved. *Rectal infection* occurs in both sexes and recent reports have described a 5–10 per cent carriage rate of gonococci in the *throat*. *Gonococcal ophthalmia*, an acute conjunctivitis in the newborn, may result from infection of the baby during birth and metastatic infections such as arthritis may be produced if the organisms invade the bloodstream. Gonococcal vulvo-vaginitis in young girls is now an uncommon infection except in association with sexual offences.

Laboratory diagnosis

The best specimens from the female are a urethral swab and a cervical swab. High and low vaginal swabs give inferior results. A swab of urethral discharge and of any discharge after prostatic massage is taken from males and rectal swabs and throat swabs may also be obtained. If possible cultures should be taken directly from the patient using a wire loop because the gonococcus is a delicate organism and dies quickly outside the body; alternatively, transport media may be used.

Although the appearance of *intracellular Gram-negative diplococci* from such specimens is virtually diagnostic of gonorrhoea, cultures are essential for medico-legal purposes. Chocolate agar, Thayer-Martin and New York City media incubated in 5–10 per cent carbon dioxide may be used. The *oxidase test* and *sugar fermentation tests* are used for further identification of suspected organisms in pure culture. *Fluorescent tests* for the identification of gonococci in smears may be used but cultural and biochemical confirmation is still required.

The gonococcal complement fixation test (GCFT) may be done but is of limited value because the gonococcus is not strongly antigenic. False-negative and false-positive reactions are common; the main problem is that of cross reactions with antibody to other commensal neisseriae.

Treatment

The gonococcus is sensitive to a wide range of antibiotics although in recent years a marked increase in resistance to penicillin has occurred. Cotrimoxazole and erythromycin are alternative drugs.

Syphilis

Bacterial aetiology

Treponema pallidum.

Pathogenesis and epidemiology

Almost all cases are contracted by sexual intercourse because like the gonococcus the causative organism is delicate and dies off rapidly outside the body. The spirochaetes present in the superficial genital lesions are passed from one partner to another through intact or damaged mucosae. When the spirochaetes have established themselves at the point of entrance they multiply rapidly and within the next three months the '*primary sore*' or '*chancre*' appears, usually on the genitalia. Although the lesion is localised the spirochaetes are distributed widely throughout the body.

The *secondary stage* occurs several weeks after clinical infection and widespread skin rashes and other lesions may occur, such as the characteristic throat and mouth ulcers and condylomata of the anus and vulva. These mucosal lesions discharge large numbers of spirochaetes. About this time the primary chancre disappears leaving only a trace of its presence, as a scar.

The *tertiary stage* is generally delayed for many years and takes the form of chronic granulomata known as *gummata*, in the brain, bone, skin and internal organs. Late manifestations of syphilis are degeneration of the brain cells producing *general paralysis of the insane* (GPI) and destruction of nerve fibres in the spinal cord causing *tabes dorsalis*. Lesions of tertiary syphilis contain few spirochaetes. The massive tissue damage may be accounted for by a delayed hypersensitivity reaction.

Laboratory diagnosis

The organisms cannot be cultivated on artifical culture media. The diagnosis of syphilis is confirmed either by finding *Treponema pallidum* in lesions or by demonstrating antibodies in the serum.

1. *Demonstration of Treponema pallidum*

Exudate from primary or secondary lesions may be examined by dark-ground microscopy. Although non-pathogenic spirochaetes may be present they are thicker and more irregular in shape, and more motile.

2. *Serological tests*

a. *Detection of antibodies against cardiolipin*. Antibodies against cardiolipin can be demonstrated by *complement fixation* as in the *Wassermann Reaction*, or by *precipitation (flocculation) tests* such as the *Kahn* and *Venereal Diseases Research Laboratory (VDRL)* tests. The latter test is simple and reliable and is now widely used.

These tests are non-specific and false-positive reactions can therefore occur, such as in pregnancy, malaria, glandular fever and in the acute stages of some infectious diseases.

b. *Detection of anti-treponemal antibody*. The Reiter protein complement fixation test (RPCF) resembles the Wassermann reaction but the antigen consists of a protein extracted from Reiter's strain of non-pathogenic spirochaetes. This is a simple test and is a very useful screening procedure.

3. *Treponema-pallidum-specific tests*

The tests that utilise *Treponema pallidum* (Nichol's strain) as an antigen are (1) the *Treponema pallidum immobilisation test (TPI)*; (2) the *fluorescent treponemal antibody absorbed test (FTA-ABS)*; and (3) the *Treponema pallidum haemagglutination test (TPHA)*.

The *TPI* test, often negative in primary syphilis, is complicated and technically difficult to perform and is used in only a few reference laboratories. The *FTA* test is simple and specific. It is generally used as a reference test when screening tests give divergent results, and is highly specific. The *TPHA* test is suitable for routine screening because it is simple to perform and commercial reagents are available. It is a very useful test although often negative in early untreated primary syphilis.

The *VDRL, RPCF* and *TPHA* tests are the most useful in routine service laboratories.

Treatment

Penicillin in high doses is very effective against *Treponema pallidum*. Erythromycin or tetracyclines may also be used in cases of penicillin hypersensitivity.

FURTHER READING

Cruickshank, R., Duguid, J. P., Marmion, B. P. & Swain, R. H. A. (1973) *Medical Microbiology*. Edinburgh: Churchill Livingstone.

Garrod, L. P., Lambert, H. P. & O'Grady, F. (1975) *Antibiotic and Chemotherapy*. Edinburgh: Churchill Livingstone.

Nicol, C. S. (1971) Gynaecology in general practice. *British Medical Journal*, 2, 328–329; 448–449; 507–509.

Walker, J., MacGillivray, I. & Macnaughton, M. C. (1976) *Combined Textbook of Obstetrics and Gynaecology*. Edinburgh: Churchill Livingstone.

Young, H., Henrichsen, C. & Robertson, D. H. H. (1974) *British Journal of Venereal Diseases*, **50**, 341–346.

13

Infections of wounds, burns and skin

Normal flora of skin

What constitutes 'normal' and what constitutes 'transient' flora is frequently difficult to establish. On the body average of two square metres of skin the various areas support different densities and species of organisms. The factors that determine selective localisation are far from clear. Different methods of sampling such as tape-stripping, scraping the *stratum corneum*, rubbing the skin with swabs and taking nutrient agar block impressions of the skin, can produce great differences in the composition and number of organisms. Three main factors determine the ecology of skin bacteria: (1) the micro climate and environment including temperature and humidity; (2) the effect of free fatty acids, other bacterial inhibitors and the low hydration of the *stratum corneum* in preventing colonisation by transient bacteria; and (3) maintenance of equilibrium of the resident flora by products of skin secretions.

The axillae, perineum and the scalp, areas of high humidity are densely colonised; the majority of the organisms reside in the superficial layers of the epidermal *stratum corneum*, although some 20 per cent of organisms reside in the deep parts of the follicular canals which are the reservoirs that re-establish the skin flora when the surface has been cleared. All people disperse bacteria on particles of desquamated skin to a greater or lesser degree but some are described as 'dangerous shedders' or 'dispersers', particularly of *Staphylococcus aureus*, and are important from the point of view of cross infection. Except for the areas mentioned the general density of bacteria on the skin is not great.

The most common bacteria of the skin are as follows: coagulase-negative and coagulase-positive staphylococci; *Sarcina* spp; lipophilic, non-lipophilic and anaerobic diphtheroids; Gram-negative bacilli (in children) and various streptococci. Nutrients for these bacteria are derived from: (1) apocrine and eccrine sweat; (2) the *stratum corneum* whose water-soluble fraction contains amino acids and peptides; and (3) fatty acids from the sebaceous glands that form the main part of skin surface lipids. Water is of prime importance and the most densely populated areas are high in humidity; dry skin supports far fewer bacteria than moist skin.

The flora of the *scalp* (hair as well as skin) differs from that of other areas because the hair produces greater humidity and higher temperatures; it has in addition a rich sebaceous gland activity. *Staphylococcus aureus*, viridans streptococci, actinomycetes and coliform organisms can all be isolated from hair.

Defences against infection

These include the intact skin, bacteriocins, lysozyme in sweat and sebum, IgA and other inhibitors. The free fatty acids derived from hydrolysis of sebum triglycerides may be bacteriocidal or bacteriostatic, although in some instances they can also be stimulatory by providing nutritional factors.

Potential pathogens (see Table 13.1)

Table 13.1 Potential pathogens of skin

Bacteria	
Staphylococcus aureus	Impetigo, Ritter's Disease (toxic epidermal necrolysis), folliculitis, furunculosis, carbuncle, ecthyma, sycosis barbae
Beta-haemolytic streptococcus	Impetigo, erysipelas, cellulitis, pemphigus
Erysipelothrix rhusiopathiae	Erysipeloid
Corynebacterium diphtheriae } *Corynebacterium ulcerans* }	Cutaneous diphtheria
Corynebacterium acnes	Acne
Mycobacterium tuberculosis	Lupus vulgaris
Mycobacterium balnei	Swimming pool granuloma
Mycobacterium ulcerans } *Mycobacterium marinum* }	Atypical cutaneous tuberculosis
Mycobacterium leprae	Leprosy
Bacillus anthracis	Anthrax (malignant pustule)
Haemophilus ducreyi	Chancroid
Treponemata	Syphilis, Yaws
Viruses	
Herpes simplex	Cold sore, herpetic whitlow
Varicella zoster	Shingles, chicken pox
Papova virus	Common wart, plantar wart
Pox viruses	Molluscum contagiosum, orf, smallpox, contagious pustular dermatitis
Coxsackie A virus	Hand, foot and mouth disease

Table 13.1 Potential pathogens of skin

Fungi	
Candida albicans	Cutaneous candidiasis
Microsporum canis *Microsporum audouinii* *Microsporum gypseum*	Scalp ringworm (Tinea capitis)
Trichophyton rubrum *Epidermophyton floccosum*	Tinea pedis
Trichophyton schoenleinii	Favus
Cryptococcus neoformans	
Actinomyces israelii	Actinomycosis
Nocardia madurae	Mycetoma (madura foot)
Protozoa	
Leishmania tropica	Tropical sore
Leishmania brasiliensis	Espundia
Metazoa	
Sarcoptes scabei	Scabies
Lice Fleas	Head, body, pubic region

Infectious diseases

Many specific infectious diseases have skin manifestations that are important features of the diseases. These include:

Bacterial infections
Meningococcaemia (*Neisseria meningitidis*)
Scarlet fever (beta-haemolytic streptococcus)

Viral infections
Rubella
Measles
Glandular fever (EB Virus)
ECHO virus infections
Chicken pox and Smallpox (see above)

Rickettsial (etc.) infections
Spotted fevers (*Rickettsia* species)

Infection of wounds

Bacterial aetiology

Many bacteria are associated with wound infection including *Staphylococcus aureus*, beta-haemolytic streptococci, *Escherichia coli*, *Proteus* spp, *Pseudomonas aeruginosa*, *Bacteroides* spp, *Clostridium welchii*, *Clostridium tetani* and anaerobic cocci. Mixed infections are common.

Pathogenesis and epidemiology

Infection may occur following trauma, injections, bites and surgery.

By far the most common wound infections are those occurring in hospitals after surgical procedures. Wound sepsis is the result of cross infection from human sources and from inanimate reservoirs. The skin and anterior nares are the most likely sources of staphylococci, the most frequent cause of wound infection; and spread occurs by the direct and indirect airborne routes and by contact. In a busy surgical ward bacterial counts per cubic feet of air (measured using slit samplers and sedimentation plates) rise during activities such as bed making and ward cleaning and fall when the ward is quiet. When a person moves about the numbers of airborne particles increase, partly because of the shedding of fresh particles from his body but also by raising particles that had fallen to the ground, and it is therefore very important to ensure that wards are not overcrowded and that hustle and bustle, particularly in the operating theatre, is kept to a minimum. Wound sepsis rates vary according to the type of surgical procedure performed, the size of the wound and the duration of the operation. Other factors such as the patient's age and general health, whether or not antibiotics are used and the efficiency of the post-operative care of the wound, all influence the sepsis rate.

Laboratory diagnosis

Pus is more satisfactory than a swab for this.

Prophylaxis

This depends on recognising the likely sources and reservoirs of infection both human and inanimate. Sources may be cases or carriers, staff or patient, and infection can be transmitted in the ward as well as in the theatre. Inanimate reservoirs include non-sterile equipment, bed linen and ward dust, and common reasons for infection are inadequate resources (for example, lack of dressing rooms), inexperienced staff, failure of aseptic techniques and failure to observe simple rules of hygiene.

Prophylaxis of wound infection depends on constant and careful surveillance of the ward and theatre environment, appraisal of sterilisation and aseptic techniques, nursing and medical procedures, and bacteriological monitoring of theatre and ward staff.

Management

When several cases of infection occur simultaneously or if the level of infection is generally at an unacceptably high level, simple epidemiological surveys and bacteriological searches for a source should be conducted. The most important act is to deal with the source if apparent. If this is a patient, isolation in a special cubicle or sideroom may be necessary and antibiotic treatment may be required. Staff who are infected should be kept away from the theatre and wards and treated. A *ward sepsis book* should be kept and close liaison with the laboratory should be maintained. An *Infection Control Officer*, often a Nursing Sister, is invaluable in such studies. Data required in the book include dates of admission, operation and onset of sepsis, type of operation and staff involved, theatre and ward involved, organisms isolated and antibiograms obtained. Such information may well pinpoint a particular individual, a break-down in some procedure, inadequate antiseptic and aseptic measures or faulty techniques. Phage typing, for example of *Staphylococcus aureus*, will indicate whether an epidemic strain is prevalent or whether the outbreaks are due to a number of other factors that can be remedied and more strictly controlled in the future.

Infection of burns

Bacterial aetiology

Organisms that colonise burns are derived mainly from the skin, upper respiratory tract and intestine of humans and include staphylococci, micrococci, streptococci, coliform organisms and corynebacteria, although environmental bacteria such as aerobic spore-bearing bacilli may also be involved. The most important pathogens are those usually acquired by cross infection such as *Pseudomonas aeruginosa*, *Staphylococcus aureus* and beta-haemolytic streptococci, groups A, B, C and G. Gram-negative bacilli are also involved, and the flora of burns is usually mixed. Anaerobes play little part in infective complications of burns.

Pathogenesis and epidemiology

Any burn not given specific prophylaxis will become colonised by bacteria within 24 hours. Colonisation may lead to local sepsis with either cellulitis in the tissues next to the burn, or septicaemia. The necrotic surface of a burn with its concomitant moisture is a good culture medium in which the bacteria can multiply, out of reach of the body's natural defences. The levels of immunoglobulin are decreased for a few days after burning.

Before separation of the slough Gram-negative bacilli tend to predominate, whereas Gram-positive organisms and fungi such as *Candida* are predominant later in the granulation tissue. The presence of beta-haemolytic streptococci is always serious as they usually prevent the take of skin grafts. Invasion by these is rare however; invasive infections are generally caused by *Pseudomonas aeruginosa*. Superficial burns are not greatly harmed by colonisation but this is not so with the deep dermal burn.

Laboratory diagnosis
Specimens of necrotic material and swabs are processed on nutrient and blood agar, aerobically and anaerobically and in cooked-meat broth. Blood cultures are essential.

Prophylaxis
Because of the frequent failure of chemotherapy and the high mortality rate in severe burns *prophylaxis* is of paramount importance. Primary excision of dead tissue and closure of the wound is beneficial in preventing infection and the application of *topical antimicrobial agents* has been shown to reduce the colonisation rates of bacteria and subsequent infection. Agents used include silver nitrate solution, chlorhexidine cream and silver sulphadiazine cream, although the use of the latter causes a great increase in resistance of Gram-negative bacilli to sulphonamides. Antibiotics may be given systemically but are not always effective. Prophylaxis with immunoglobulin may be of use where topical chemoprophylaxis is difficult.

Infections of the skin and subcutaneous tissues

Acne
Bacterial aetiology. Corynebacterium acnes, anaerobic diphtheroids, coagulase-negative staphylococci and micrococci are associated with this condition.

Pathogenesis. Diffusible products of certain organisms may produce acne and the role of free fatty acids may be of importance.

Treatment. Many forms have been attempted. The role of antibiotics is questionable; *in vitro* testing does not identify an effective antibiotic, although some success is claimed for tetracyclines.

Bacterial infections of the skin

Staphylococcal infections
Boils or furuncles are the most common lesions caused by *Staphylococcus aureus*. These infections are circumscribed, with suppurative central necrosis which eventually discharges as a small slough with pus. A *blind boil* subsides without discharge of pus. A

carbuncle is a large abscess, much more serious than a boil, that occurs at the back of the neck in the thick collagenous tissues. It is a laterally-burrowing subcutaneous infection in which there are multiple openings to the skin, and it occurs most commonly in diabetics. *Staphylococcus aureus* also causes *breast abscess* in nursing mothers, and other superficial lesions that include *sycosis barbae* (face), *blepharitis* (eyelid), *stye* (eyelash follicle) and *conjunctivitis.* (Conjunctivitis is also caused by *Haemophilus influenzae* and *Streptococcus pneumoniae*). A form of *ecthyma, bullous impetigo* and *toxic epidermal necrolysis* are all caused by *Staphylococcus aureus.*

Streptococcal infections

These are mostly caused by *Streptococcus pyogenes* and include *cellulitis,* a spreading infection of the subcutaneous tissues and *erysipelas,* a similar infection of the dermis. In the latter, lesions occur on the limbs and on the face where the typical butterfly rash (cheek-nose-cheek) is seen. Repeated attacks of this infection are possible and may be due to the manifestation of a hypersensitivity reaction to the streptococci rather than to direct infection. Streptococcal *ecthyma* and *impetigo* also occur. This form of impetigo is less common than staphylococcal and is clinically different in that the lesions are yellow, typically discrete and subsequently form crusts. *Scarlet fever* is also associated with streptococcal infection, usually of the throat.

Gram-negative infections

Gram-negative organisms are rare on healthy skin except in moist areas such as the groin and axilla. *Proteus* spp are common in the latter site and this is thought to be due to the use of underarm deodorants. Coliform organisms and *Bacteroides* spp may be isolated from abscesses, particularly in the area between the thighs and the waist, and may be related to preceding trauma. *Pseudomonas aeruginosa* may be involved in chronic paronychia generally in association with *Candida* spp.

Miscellaneous infections

One of the commonest infections, *trichomycosis axillaris,* is caused by overgrowth of diphtheroids on the shaft of axillary hairs and can lead to sweat discoloration of clothing. *Erysipeloid* is an infection of the hands and fingers caused by *Erysipelothrix rhusiopathiae,* and is an occupational hazard for those who handle infected animals or fish. Other infections include *syphilis* (Ch. 12), *anthrax* and *leprosy* (Ch. 14).

FURTHER READING

Davidson, A. I. G., Smylie, H. G., Macdonald, A. & Smith, G. (1971) Ward design in relation to postoperative wound infection. *British Medical Journal*, **1**, 72–75.

Gibson, G. L. (1974) *Infection in Hospital*. Edinburgh: Churchill Livingstone.

Lowbury, E. J. L., Ayliffe, G. A. J., Geddes, A. M. & Williams, J. P. (1975) *Control of Hospital Infection: A Practical Handbook*. London: Chapman and Hall.

Lowbury, E. J. L. (1976) Prophylaxis and treatment for infection of burns. *British Journal of Hospital Medicine*, **15**, 566–572.

Marks, R. & Samman, P. D. (1977) *Dermatology*. London: Heinemann.

Noble, W. C. (1971). Microbial skin disease. *British Journal of Dermatology*, **86**, Suppl. 8.

Noone, P. & Griffiths, R. J. (1971) The effect on sepsis rates of closing and cleaning hospital wards. *Journal of Clinical Pathology*, **24**, 721–725.

Parker, M. T. & Williams, R. E. O. (1961) Further observations on the bacteriology of impetigo and pemphigus neonatorum. *Acta Paediatrica*, **50**, 101–112.

Selwyn, S. (1965) The mechanism and prevention of cross-infection in dermatological wards. *Journal of Hygiene*, **63**, 59–71.

Smylie, H. G., Davidson, A. I. G., Macdonald, A. & Smith, G. (1971) Ward design in relation to postoperative wound infection. *British Medical Journal*, **1**, 67–72.

Williams, R. E. O., Blowers, R., Garrod, L. P. & Shooter, R. A. (1966) *Hospital Infection: Causes and prevention*. London: Lloyd-Luke.

14

Miscellaneous bacterial infections

Actinomycosis

Bacterial aetiology

In man the principal infecting organism is *Actinomyces israelii*. *Actinomyces naeslundii* may also be involved and *Actinomyces bovis* produces actinomycosis in cattle.

Pathogenesis and epidemiology

Actinomycosis can occur in the lung and ileo-caecal region but by far the most common areas are the face and neck. It is an uncommon, chronic suppurative and granulomatous infection with sinus formation and discharge of pus containing *'sulphur granules'* that are colonies of *Actinomyces*. *Actinomyces israelii* is a normal inhabitant of the mouth. Infection of the cervicofacial region occurs by local invasion and may follow trauma such as fracture of the jaw and tooth extraction, or it may be due to the presence of teeth with gangrenous pulps.

Laboratory diagnosis

Pus must be examined for the presence of granules which if present should be crushed, and a Gram film made. Granules consist of Gram-positive branching filaments with Gram-negative clubbed ends, which on tissue section can be seen to radiate from a central mass of mycelium. Cultures are made on blood agar incubated anaerobically for four to seven days. Further fermentation tests are required for identification.

Treatment

Penicillin is the most appropriate drug in addition to necessary surgical measures. A six-week course of treatment is recommended. Tetracycline is an alternative drug.

Anthrax

Bacterial aetiology
Bacillus anthracis.

Pathogenesis and epidemiology
Anthrax, a zoonosis, is a septicaemic infection of herbivora, mainly sheep and cattle, although virtually all animals are susceptible to some degree. The disease is uncommon in the United Kingdom and outbreaks that occur, for example in zoos, are due to ingestion of spores in contaminated foodstuffs. Human anthrax is uncommon and occurs by contact or inhalation in people dealing with animals or products of animals that have died from the disease, for example shaving brushes, wool, skins, bones and bone meal, hair and bristles. Two forms of human anthrax occur, cutaneous infection, *malignant pustule*, and very rarely a haemorrhagic infection of the lung, *woolsorters' disease*.

Laboratory diagnosis
Vesicular fluid or swabs from a suspected malignant pustule should be examined for large Gram-positive bacilli; these are virtually diagnostic. Various cultural features such as characteristic colonies and non-motility distinguish anthrax bacilli from other sporing bacilli, but pathogenicity tests on mice or guinea pigs are essential for confirmation of identity.

Prophylaxis
Animals may be immunised against anthrax. Infected animals must be killed and cremated or buried deeply. Rigid control of importation of hides and protection of the hands and other exposed skin surfaces of workers have reduced the incidence of the disease.

Treatment
Penicillin is the drug of choice but may not be effective in the serious respiratory form.

Brucellosis

Bacterial aetiology
Three main species of *Brucella* occur in different animal hosts:

Brucella abortus:	Cattle
Brucella melitensis:	Goats and sheep
Brucella suis:	Pigs

Pathogenesis and epidemiology

Each of the three species is pathogenic to man. *Brucella abortus* is the commonest in the United Kingdom. The organisms produce contagious abortion in cattle and then localise in the mammary glands. Uterine discharges, urine, faeces and milk may all contain the bacilli and human infections occur by handling infected carcases, by contact with infected discharges, or by drinking infected milk or milk products. Infection can be contracted through abrasions in the skin and through the alimentary and conjunctival mucosae. Human brucellosis occurs predominantly in farmers, veterinary workers and in those who drink unpasteurised milk but as it is a zoonosis there is no man-to-man spread.

The bacteria localise and multiply inside the cells of the reticulo-endothelial system forming granulomatous lesions in the liver and spleen where they are inaccessible to the circulating phagocytes. Clinically the disease may be acute, subacute or chronic. Subclinical infections also occur and these are common in veterinary surgeons.

Laboratory diagnosis

Repeated *blood cultures* should be taken, although they are often negative in the disease, and they should be incubated in an atmosphere of 5–10 per cent carbon dioxide for three to four weeks before being discarded. Castaneda's method using a bottle that contains solid and fluid media may be useful. After isolation species differentiation depends on biochemical tests.

Serological tests are helpful in the second week of clinical infection, as both agglutinating (IgM) antibodies and complement-fixing (IgG) antibodies are present in the acute stage. In chronic brucellosis IgM antibodies decrease and may be absent even when the patient is clinically ill.

Antiglobulin tests (Coombs' test) can also be done.

Prophylaxis

Animals must be tested and positive reactors slaughtered or segregated. It is possible to vaccinate animals, for example female calves, against the disease but because of undesirable side effects this is not recommended for man. A milk ring test (MRT) is used to screen for infection in dairy cattle. Pasteurisation of milk has also helped reduce the incidence of the disease.

Therapy

Many antibiotics are effective in acute and subacute infections, particularly a combination of oral tetracycline and intramuscular streptomycin. Chemotherapy has nothing to offer in the treatment of chronic infection.

Gas gangrene

Bacterial aetiology

Clostridium welchii (*perfringens*) is the main organism involved. Others include *Clostridium oedematiens* (*novyi*), *septicum*, *histolyticum* and the *bifermentans-sordellii* group.

Pathogenesis and epidemiology

Gas gangrene is caused as the result of toxin production by clostridia and occurs when there is damaged or devitalised tissue which will provide the required conditions for anaerobic growth. *Clostridium welchii* and other clostridia can normally be isolated from human and animal faeces and their spores are ubiquitous in nature. They can be isolated from the skin of the perineum and thighs and when gas gangrene results from surgical intervention in these areas it is usually an endogenous infection. This type of infection is seen in older patients following mid-thigh amputations for ischaemic disease of the lower limbs. Three types of wound infection are recognised: (1) *simple contamination* of wounds where the organisms do no harm, the commonest type of presentation; (2) *Clostridial cellulitis*, an acute, spreading infection of the subcutaneous tissues; and (3) *Clostridial myositis*, or true gas gangrene in which muscles are invaded; septicaemia and toxaemia are common.

Laboratory diagnosis

Gram-stained films demonstrate large Gram-positive bacilli and anaerobic blood agar cultures yield heavy growths of clostridia. Toxin production should be investigated.

Prophylaxis

Surgical removal of devitalised tissue is the basis of prophylaxis. When surgical procedures are to be carried out in the area of the thigh, perineum and buttocks, particularly in the elderly, prophylactic penicillin should be administered.

Treatment

Removal of devitalised tissue is again required as well as large doses of antibiotic, preferably penicillin. Hyperbaric oxygen therapy can be given in addition to polyvalent antitoxic serum.

Leprosy

Bacterial aetiology
Mycobacterium leprae.

Pathogenesis and epidemiology
The organism is a human parasite that cannot be made to infect laboratory animals by conventional methods, although experimental infection of the mouse foot pad is possible. The infectivity of the disease is low and requires long and close contact; it is probably contracted both through skin abrasions and also by inhalation of infected dust. It is now mainly confined to tropical countries such as Ethiopia.

Leprosy is a chronic granulomatous infection. In the *lepromatous* and *nodular* types granulomata form in the skin, mucosae and various organs. In the *tuberculoid* type there is infiltration of certain motor and sensory nerves.

Laboratory diagnosis
This depends on demonstrating acid-fast bacilli in smears and tissue scrapings. The organisms resemble *Mycobacterium tuberculosis* and bacteria are commonly seen inside mononuclear lepra cells. The organisms cannot be grown on artificial media.

Prophylaxis
Vaccination has been recommended particularly against tuberculoid leprosy, but further studies are required to confirm the usefulness of this. Health education is also important.

Treatment
Oral sulphones, clofazimine or rifampicin may be used.

Leptospiral infections

(a) **Weil's disease**

Bacterial aetiology
Leptospira icterohaemorrhagiae.

Pathogenesis and epidemiology
The organisms which produce leptospirosis, a zoonosis, are normally carried in the kidneys of the brown rat. They cause no harm to the rats, but are excreted in their urine usually for life; they can live for days in stagnant water, mud and moist earth, and infection occurs

through abrasions in the skin and mucous membranes. Agricultural workers, miners, fish handlers and sewer workers are all liable to infection but leptospirosis can also be caused by drinking infected water or bathing in canals, ponds or rivers. Leptospires multiply in the bloodstream and spread tò the liver, kidneys and lungs, which accounts for the *protean manifestations* of the disease. They have a particular predilection for the kidney cortex where they colonise the convoluted tubules and remain there for some time.

(b) **Canicola fever**

Bacterial aetiology
Leptospira canicola.

Pathogenesis and epidemiology
Another leptospiral serotype causes this disease which often presents as meningitis, with particularly severe headache and conjunctivitis. Puppies are prone to canicola fever. Children contract it from the infected excreta of a sick puppy, particularly one with nephritis, Pigs are also commonly infected.

Laboratory diagnosis of leptospiral infections
After an incubation period of five to twelve days leptospires may be seen in the blood by dark-ground microscopy and in the second week of the infection they may be seen in the urine. Guinea-pig inoculation of body fluids may be useful, and special media for blood and urine culture are available. Serological tests are useful as antibodies are detectable from the end of the first week; agglutination tests and complement fixation tests are widely used.

Prophylaxis
Education of dog owners is important and workers at risk should wear suitable protective clothing. Puppies should be immunised. Prophylactic vaccination is also given to certain groups of workers where the risk is high.

Treatment
Leptospirosis may be treated by penicillin which is the drug of choice. Tetracyclines are alternative agents, although in general antibiotics are only effective in influencing the course of the disease if they are given in the first week of the illness.

Plague

Bacterial aetiology
Yersinia pestis.

Pathogenesis and epidemiology
The plague bacillus is a parasite of rodents (particularly rats) and their fleas spread infection to other animals. Infected rats living around human habitation are commonly responsible for outbreaks of human plague and the infection is spread to man by infected rat fleas. Man-to-man infection is rare except from a patient with *pneumonic plague* who may disperse infected droplets in the environment. In *bubonic plague* lymph nodes are affected, in particular those draining the area of the flea bite. Glands (buboes) swell in the groin, axilla or neck depending on the site of the bite. Septicaemia and death may thereafter occur. In *pneumonic plague* the patient suffers from a severe haemorrhagic bronchopneumonia. The virulence of the plague bacillus relates to factors that protect it from phagocytosis, such as capsular and somatic antigens.

Laboratory diagnosis
Diagnosis is confirmed by isolation of bacilli from buboes or sputum. The bacilli show characteristic bipolar staining with methylene blue. Blood cultures may yield the organism and should be taken in suspected cases. Isolation on blood agar is facilitated by anaerobic conditions at 27°C. Inoculation of pathological material on to the nasal mucosa of guinea pigs or rats may yield the pure cultures necessary for biochemical identification.

Prophylaxis
This essentially means control over wild and domestic rat populations and particularly fleas if epidemics threaten. Vaccination can provide immunity of short duration.

Treatment
Large doses of tetracycline are recommended for both bubonic and pneumonic plague.

Rat-bite fever

Bacterial aetiology
Spirillum minus and *Streptobacillus moniliformis* produce diseases that

are clinically indistinguishable. Both organisms can be isolated from the respiratory tract of rats.

Pathogenesis and epidemiology

Rat-bite fever is a relapsing febrile illness with local inflammation at the site of the bite, enlargement of local lymph glands and a macular skin eruption. A multiple arteritis may occur. *Spirillum minus* infection occurs in Japan and the Far East whereas *Streptobacillus moniliformis* infection occurs in the Americas.

Spirillum minus can be demonstrated by dark-ground illumination in fresh preparations of lesions or lymph glands and also in the blood of mice or guinea pigs 10 days after injection. The organisms can be stained by Leishman's stain or by ordinary aniline dyes, but as they cannot be cultured on inanimate media some workers class them as spirochaetes. Spirilla differ from these however in that they are rigid and owe their motility to polar flagella.

Streptobacillus moniliformis. These organisms can be isolated from blood cultures and from fluid media that have a high content of blood, serum or ascitic fluid. They are highly pleomorphic and L forms occur.

Treatment

Both forms respond well to penicillin, and tetracycline is active against L forms of *Streptobacillus moniliformis.*

Relapsing fever

Bacterial aetiology

The causative organisms are *Borrelia recurrentis,* the infecting organism of European (louse-borne) relapsing fever, and *Borrelia duttonii,* the infecting organism of African (tick-borne) relapsing fever.

Pathogenesis and epidemiology

Louse-borne fever may be endemic or epidemic in conditions of cold and overcrowding. After lice become infected they cannot transmit infection for a few days; the multiplying spirochaetes then enter the coelomic cavity. Coelomic fluid of infected crushed lice or infected excreta may enter the human through abrasions. Bouts of fever lasting from two to four days are separated by intervals of around one week. Many relapses can occur and it is thought that each relapse is produced by fresh antigenic types of organisms. Wild rodents are the principal sources of infection with *Borrelia duttonii.* Human cases result from tick bites or contamination of wounds with infected secretions. The organisms persist throughout the life of the tick and are transferred to succeeding generations through the ova. Unlike louse-borne fever, tick-borne fever does not occur epidemically.

Laboratory diagnosis

This is made by the demonstration of borreliae in blood films stained by Giemsa's or Leishman's methods or dilute carbol fuchsin, particularly during pyrexial phases. Dark-ground microscopy of blood is also useful. Inoculation of rats produces considerable numbers of borreliae in their blood within 48 hours.

Treatment

Tetracyclines, penicillin and chloramphenicol are all effective in the treatment of these infections.

FURTHER READING

Christie, A. B. (1974) *Infectious Diseases: Epidemiology and Clinical Practice*. Edinburgh: Churchill Livingstone.

Cruickshank, R., Duguid, J. P., Marmion, B. P. & Swain, R. H. A. (1973) *Medical Microbiology*. Edinburgh: Churchill Livingstone.

Dubos, R. J. & Hirsch, J. G. (1965) *Bacterial and Mycotic Infections of Man*. London: Pitman.

Henderson, R. J. & Hill, D. M. (1972) Subclinical brucella infection in man. *British Medical Journal*, **3**, 154–6.

Lamb, R. (1973) Anthrax. *British Medical Journal*, **1**, 157–159.

Lawson, J. H. (1971) Leptospirosis. *British Journal of Hospital Medicine*, 5, 357–364.

Welsby, P. D. & Smith, C. C. (1978) Brucellosis: the current position. *British Journal of Hospital Medicine*, **19**, 20–27.

Index